CPD for Non-Medical Prescribers

A Practical Guide

Edited by

Marion Waite and Jan Keenan

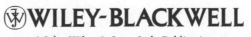
WILEY-BLACKWELL

A John Wiley & Sons, Ltd., Publication

This edition first published 2010
© 2010 by Blackwell Publishing Ltd

Blackwell Publishing was acquired by John Wiley & Sons in February 2007.
Blackwell's publishing programme has been merged with Wiley's global Scientific, Technical, and Medical business to form Wiley-Blackwell.

Registered office
John Wiley & Sons Ltd, The Atrium, Southern Gate, Chichester, West Sussex, PO19 8SQ, United Kingdom

Editorial offices
9600 Garsington Road, Oxford, OX4 2DQ, United Kingdom
2121 State Avenue, Ames, Iowa 50014-8300, USA

For details of our global editorial offices, for customer services and for information about how to apply for permission to reuse the copyright material in this book please see our website at http://www.wiley.com/wiley-blackwell.

The right of the author to be identified as the author of this work has been asserted in accordance with the UK Copyright, Designs and Patents Act 1988.

Library of Congress Cataloging-in-Publication Data
CPD for non-medical prescribers : a practical guide / edited by Marion Waite and Jan Keenan.
        p. ; cm.
   Includes bibliographical references and index.
   ISBN 978-1-4051-7885-3 (pbk. : alk. paper) 1. Nurses – Prescription privileges – Great Britain. 2. Drugs – Prescribing – Great Britain. 3. Medicine – Study and teaching (Continuing education) – Great Britain. I. Waite, Marion. II. Keenan, Jan. III. Title: Continuing professional development for non-medical prescribers.
   [DNLM: 1. Education, Pharmacy – methods – Great Britain. 2. Clinical Competence – Great Britain. 3. Drug Prescriptions – standards – Great Britain. 4. Education, Continuing – methods – Great Britain. QV 20 C882 2010]
   RT81.8.C63 2010
   610.73 – dc22

                                                          2009024678

A catalogue record for this book is available from the British Library.

Typeset in 10/12.5 Palatino by Laserwords Private Limited, Chennai, India
Printed and bound in Malaysia by KHL Printing Co Sdn Bhd

1   2010

Contents

List of Contributors

Sanjay Desai
MRPharmS, Dip Com Pharm, MSc,
Independent and Supplementary Prescriber
Pharmaceutical Adviser
Joint Non-Medical Prescribing Lead
NHS Berkshire West
Lecturer
University of Reading

Michael Fanning
RN, DPSN, MSc
Deputy Director of Nursing and Quality
Oxford Radcliffe Hospitals NHS Trust

Mandy Fry
MBBS, DCH, DFFP, MPhil, MRCGP
Portfolio GP, Cirencester & Senior Lecturer in Primary Care
Oxford Brookes University

Jan Keenan
RN, DipHE (Lond), MSc, PGDipEd
Non-Medical Prescriber Consultant Nurse
Cardiac Medicine and Joint Non-Medical Prescribing Lead
Oxford Radcliffe Hospitals NHS Trust

Dan Lasserson
MA, MBBS (Hons), MRCP(UK), MRCGP
GP Principal, Oxford Clinical Lecturer
Department of Primary Health Care
University of Oxford

Fiona Peniston-Bird
RN, RHV, BSc (Hons)
Nurse Independent Prescriber
Independent Non-Medical Prescribing Development Consultant
Lecturer Non-Medical Prescribing
University of Winchester

Anne Smith
RN, BSc (Hons) Community Health Care (D/N), MSc, PGCHE, FPT
Director of Nursing Studies
University of Reading

Nicola Stoner
BSc (Hons), MRPharmS, (SPresc & IPresc), Dip Clin Pharm, PhD, ACPP
Consultant Pharmacist
Oxford Radcliffe Hospitals NHS Trust
Honorary Principal Visiting Fellow
The School of Pharmacy
University of Reading

Marion Waite
RN, RM, RHV, BA, MSc
Community Specialist Practitioner Award
Nurse Prescriber, Practice Educator
Senior Lecturer Non-Medical Prescribing
Oxford Brookes University
Visiting Diabetes Specialist Nurse
Oxford

Acknowledgements

The editors are indebted to the following, for their kind permission to publish their examples of excellent practice:

The *Department of Health*, and in particular to *Stuart Merritt*, Non-Medical Prescribing Lead, for 'Making the Connections', work led by Yorkshire and Humberside Strategic Health Authority with contributions from the Department of Health. For further information, readers can contact *Alison Dale*, Clinical and Education Lead, Non-Medical Prescribing and Pharmacy: Alison.dale@yorksandhumber.nhs.uk

Sarah Knight, Programme Manager, JISC E-learning Programme, JISC Innovation Group, for permission to include the JISC Effective E-learning Planner.

Dr John Reynolds, Chair of the Medicines Advisory Committee, and *Olubunmi Fajemisin*, Clinical Effectiveness Pharmacist, both of the Oxford Radcliffe Hospitals NHS Trust, for the excellent Medicines Information Leaflets produced on behalf of the Committee, and for the contributions of the authors of the documents, *Fiona Singleton*, Oxfordshire Smoking Cessation Advisor and *Scott Harrison*, Lead Pharmacist, Anticoagulation.

Jane Nicholls, NHS London Non-Medical Prescribing Lead, and *Marcia Osuno* of Barking and Havering PCT, for their Clinical Governance Audit tool.

Sarah Wilds and the *Medicines Management Team of Oxfordshire PCT*, for examples of '*Prescribing Points*', a newsletter for Primary Care Trust prescribers.

Akin Adeniaran, Pharmacist and Senior Lecturer, Oxford Brookes University, for developing an example of a pharmacology self-test, included in Chapter 7.

Oxford Brookes University Library Services for their support in developing an example search strategy (see Appendix 9).

Introduction

Marion Waite and Jan Keenan

The advent of non-medical prescribing has heralded a new era for the development of the health professions. Without question, it has opened new avenues for service development, creating opportunities for developing accessibility to medications, streamlining existing services for the benefit of patients and importantly, developing and making use of the exceptional skills of health professionals.

Paradoxically, it has been greeted and embraced with both enthusiasm and scepticism. Although incorporated willingly into practice, there are some concerns that it could be a step too far. Yet, the number of non-medical prescribers within England, Scotland and Wales is estimated to be over 40,000. This includes community practitioner nurse prescribers; independent and supplementary nurse prescribers; independent and supplementary pharmacist prescribers and allied health professional supplementary prescribers including physiotherapists, podiatrists, chiropodists and radiographers.

Prescribers work in as diverse a range of specialities and contexts as the delivery of health care itself, in general practice, in the acute and continuing care sectors and in the community. One thing every prescriber has in common is a personal need and professional obligation to keep abreast of the pace of developments in health care that affect every practitioner. In January 2008, the National Prescribing Centre (NPC) undertook an online survey of new prescribers, part of which concerned the need for continuing professional development (CPD) (NPC 2008). Half of the non-medial prescribers surveyed felt that they were fully utilised, and more than half stated that their organisation did not have a structured CPD programme in place. Twenty-seven percent felt that current provision did not meet their needs. Very high on the list of priorities for what CPD programmes should cover were medicines management, drug interactions and therapeutics.

Our experience locally and nationally is that non-medical prescribers find their CPD from a variety of sources, both within and outside the workplace. What is very clear in any forum is that non-medical prescribers take the responsibility for their own CPD very seriously.

This book is a practical guide for individual non-medical prescribers, their managers, commissioners and prescribing leads at both local and regional levels, who have the responsibility for providing CPD for non-medical prescribers. The Nursing and Midwifery Council (NMC 2008) and the Royal Pharmaceutical Society of Great Britain (RPSGB 2008) have identified standards for CPD for non-medical prescribers.

This has implications for individual practitioners and the health-care organisations employing them. Each has an important role in ensuring that these standards are met. It is crucial that non-medical prescribers can ensure that they are safe, effective and competent within their prescribing roles and can further develop their prescribing practice in order to meet patient and service needs.

This book provides an accessible context that outlines the issues in relation to CPD and non-medical prescribing, including the legal and professional frameworks within which non-medical prescribers practise. It also provides practical examples of working, usable documents as well as resources to ensure that non-medical prescribers can remain up to date within the diversity of settings in which they undertake their prescribing roles. Each of these is contained either within the chapter itself or as a related key resource in a third section.

The book consists of three sections; the first consists of four chapters, each of which explores a fundamental aspect of the principles of CPD for non-medical prescribers. This section refers to overarching and organisational issues that impact on non-medical prescribing. The pace at which non-medical prescribing has developed is remarkable, and following the initial changes in the law that impacted on the development of prescribing was difficult. Subsequent to the opening up of non-medical prescribing to allow nurses and pharmacists to prescribe from the British National Formulary (BNF) rather than restricted lists of medications, there has been a slower momentum of change but it remains difficult to keep ahead of consultations and legal and professional developments. An initial chapter by Marion Waite, *Keeping Up to Date with Legal and Professional Issues* outlines the current legal and professional frameworks that support non-medical prescribing and offers a series of accessible resources and approaches for keeping up to date.

Subsequent chapters in Section One deal with organisational issues in relation to non-medical prescribing, as well as offer resources that support the organisation, the employer and the individual in accessing CPD. Anne Smith and Sanjay Desai in *Prescribing Practice from the Employers' Perspective: The Rationale for CPD within Non-medical Prescribing* outline the importance of the role of the non-medical prescribing lead within an organisation in supporting the role of non-medical prescribers as well as managing competing demands on resources. They discuss the importance of ensuring that non-medical prescribers remain safe and competent to provide a high standard of patient care.

Michael Fanning in *Developing an Organisational Non-medical Prescribing Policy that Supports Continuing Professional Development* discusses clinical governance issues in relation to prescribing, through the process of developing an organisational policy for non-medical prescribing that supports the importance of CPD. In *Organising Continuing Professional Development for Non-medical Prescribers at a Regional Level*, Fiona Peniston-Bird provides an overview of the structure of the National Health Service (NHS) in England, Scotland and Wales and how this relates to the development of the non-medical prescribing role. It includes lessons learned from networking within a national forum, and how these translate to organising CPD at a regional level.

Section Two consists of five chapters, each of which explores a different approach to facilitating CPD for non-medical prescribers. This takes into account differing learning styles, the diversity of non-medical prescribers and the accessibility to resources that may be available to support CPD. E-learning has become a feature of many formal courses, but there are significant advances in this field that support non-medical prescribers. In *Using e-Learning to Support Continuing Professional Development for Non-medical Prescribers,* Marion Waite offers a practical guide to the use of blended learning for non-medical prescribers that includes principles of designing online learning activities and the potential use of other learning technologies within an NHS organisation or Trust. The chapter is based on an evaluation project of CPD e-learning at regional NHS level as well as the practical experience of running blended learning in non-medical prescribing courses and non-medical prescribing CPD updates. A non-medical prescriber and an organisational non-medical prescribing lead, Jan Keenan has used action learning to facilitate CPD as well as organise the delivery of CPD in a large organisation as well as at speciality level. The chapter *Action Learning and Learning Sets* concerns itself with some of the theoretical aspects of action learning and, in addition, offers the benefit of experience in developing support systems for prescribers. This includes examples of how to involve non-medical prescribers in CPD activity within a busy organisation as well as how non-medical prescribers can raise the profile of service developments and the profile of non-medical prescribing as an essential component of service delivery.

Nicola Stoner presents the chapter on *Keeping Up to Date with Pharmacology,* which outlines the principles of prescribing effectively and safely. The chapter outlines the importance of keeping up to date with pharmacology within a prescribing role. All non-medical prescribers will have been introduced to general principles of pharmacology during their initial non-medical prescriber training. This acts as a revision guide for those principles and is supported by a section on techniques to support the teaching and learning of pharmacology within practice. The chapter also identifies key sources of support and advice for pharmacological or drug knowledge within practice and identifies the role of a supervisory relationship in order to support this.

Dr Mandy Fry outlines the potential opportunities for CPD for non-medical prescribers in the chapter *Organising Continuing Professional Development for Non-medical Prescribers in a General Practice Setting*. There is a particular focus on the continued importance and use of mentors for preceptorship for the newly qualified non-medical prescriber, taking into account the context of general practice and the resources and sources of support and advice, which may be accessible within this setting. Dr Dan Lasserson offers a practical guide to setting up a journal club in clinical practice and focuses on evidence-based prescribing issues. His chapter, *Organising and Running a Journal Club for Non-medical Prescribers*, also considers why evidence-based practice is important for the prescriber and outlines techniques and strategies for getting evidence into practice. The chapter additionally deals with how to get others on board and maintain momentum in the longer term.

Section Three offers key resources and practice examples for non-medical prescribers. It contains nine appendices, each of which relates to one chapter and contains usable resources in order to provide CPD for non-medical prescribers. Each appendix identifies further resources and includes some practical ideas, tools and objects, which may be transferred to a variety of settings. All of these have been drawn from examples that are currently in use at a local, regional and national level to support CPD, and each has been critically appraised for reliability and validity.

The contributors to this book are all health professionals from a variety of backgrounds, who have experience and expertise in supporting, developing or delivering CPD for non-medical prescribers and other groups of health-care professionals. Our aim has been to draw together their expertise and experience in the provision of CPD and to offer a variety of trusted and usable resources to support non-medical prescribers.

References

Nursing and Midwifery Council (2008) *Guidance for Continuing Professional Development for Nurse and Midwife Prescribers*. London. NMC.

National Prescribing Centre (NPC) (2008) *Connecting Prescribers* Issue 9; March 2008.

The Royal Pharmaceutical Society of Great Britain (RPGSB) *CPD Template* http://www.uptodate.org.uk/home/PlanRecord.shtml.

Section One

General Principles for Continuing Professional Development for Non-Medical Prescribers

1 Keeping Up to Date with Legal and Professional Frameworks for Non-Medical Prescribing

Marion Waite

Introduction

The purpose of this chapter is to consider the relevance of keeping up to date with legal and professional frameworks that govern non-medical prescribing. This has implications for both non-medical prescribers and the organisations that employ them.

Professional responsibility refers to the liability to be called to account for actions (Dimond 2008). The duty of care as a non-medical prescriber implies a responsibility to demonstrate appropriate knowledge in relation to the prescribing of drugs and medicines. This includes knowledge of the legal framework that governs the licensing, supply and administration of drugs and medicines as applied to the non-medical prescribing role. This also includes standards for professional practice, which relates to continuing professional development (CPD) and, although not legally binding, constitute best practice within non-medical prescribing.

This chapter outlines the current legal and professional frameworks for non-medical prescribing. Explicit reference will be made to significant legal changes and professional recommendations for standards for non-medical prescribing. The chapter will also consider how the non-medical prescriber can keep up to date with these aspects once qualified and the role of the employer in this process.

In our experience of running non-medical prescribing courses and providing CPD updates for non-medical prescribers, keeping up with changes in the legal and professional frameworks that underpin non-medical prescribing can be a challenging issue. This is because there have been rapid changes within these frameworks within a relatively short space of time, especially between the years 2002 and 2006.

The law as it applies to medicines

The term *law* here includes Acts of Parliament and Statutory Instruments and applies to legislation of the European Community and legislation of the state. The main legislation in the United Kingdom is the Medicines Act 1968 and the Misuse of Drugs Act 1971.

This legislation regulates the supply, storage and administration of medicines, and the purpose is to protect the public from harm. The Medicines Act 1968 is a comprehensive statute and encompasses the Medicines and Healthcare products Regulatory Agency (MHRA) which is the governmental body that oversees the licensing and safety of medicines. Furthermore the Medicines Act 1968 categorises drugs for purposes of sale and supply to the public into three groups: Pharmacy-only Products (P), General Sales List (GSL) and Prescription-only Medicines (POM).

The qualified non-medical prescriber has a duty of care to keep up to date with how these regulations are amended and with ongoing safety profiles as applied to the formulary of drugs within their sphere of competence. Timely information can be accessed from the MHRA website http://www.mhra.gov.uk/index.htm.

The British National Formulary (BNF), is a joint publication of the British Medical Association (BMA) and the Royal Pharmaceutical Society of Great Britain (RPSGB). It is published biannually and aims to provide prescribers with thorough and up to date information on the legal and clinical use of medicines, which includes medicine regulations.

The Misuse of Drugs Act 1971 lists and classifies controlled drugs and creates criminal offences in relation to the manufacture, supply and possession of controlled drugs, gives the Secretary of State the power to make regulations and directions to prevent misuse of controlled drugs and powers of search, arrest and forfeiture.

In 2001, the statutory instrument Misuse of Drug Regulations 2001 classified controlled drugs into five schedules outlining the requirements, which govern the import, export, production, supply possession, prescribing and record keeping. The non-medical prescriber has a duty of care to keep up to date with these schedules as applied to the formulary of drugs within their sphere of competence. Timely information can be accessed as an appendix of the BNF.

The law as it applies to non-medical prescribing roles

Independent prescribing

The Prescription by Nurses Act 1992 was implemented following the recommendations of the first Crown Report (DH 1989). This enabled health visitors and district nurses who had completed specific training to prescribe from a designated limited formulary of medicines. Approximately 29,000 community nurses in the United Kingdom hold this qualification. Since May 2006, this is referred to as *community practitioner nurse prescribing* and it is still possible to undertake the training as a component of the Nursing and Midwifery Council (NMC) Specialist Community Practitioner Award.

A second Crown Report (DH 1999) was commissioned in order to provide strategic and consistent direction for extending prescribing rights and responsibilities to other groups of health professionals. The report outlined the sphere of possibilities for non-medical prescribing and explored the implications for professional bodies, National Health Service (NHS) organisations, education providers and other stakeholders. Following consultation on the report, Section 63 of the Health and Social Care Act 2001 amended the Medicines Act 1968, and The NHS Act 1977 Regulations were amended (Dimond 2008) in order to allow the extension of nurse prescribing from the Extended Independent Nurse Prescribers' Formulary. This allowed nurses, midwives and health visitors who had completed specific nurse-independent extended prescribing training to prescribe a limited range of drugs licensed to explicit medical conditions categorised under four headings: minor illness, minor injuries, palliative care and health promotion.

Following a number of incremental changes to increase the range of drugs and medical conditions, the Extended Independent Nurse Prescribers' Formulary became defunct on 1 May 2006 owing to the implementation of the Independent Prescribing (IP) Regulations 2006. This enables nurses, midwives, health visitors and pharmacists who have completed specific IP training to prescribe any licensed medicine (including private prescriptions) for any medical condition that the practitioner is competent to treat. This also includes a limited range of borderline substances and off-label prescribing where it constitutes best practice. For nurses, midwives and health visitors this also includes a limited range of controlled drugs where appropriate.

In 2007, further amendments enabled optometrists to prescribe licensed medicine (including private prescriptions) for any medical condition that the practitioner is competent to treat.

In July 2009 the MHRA announced that further legal changes would take place by the end of 2009 to enable independent nurse prescribers to prescribe unlicensed medicines where this constitutes best practice to treat any condition.

Responsibility for accrediting training courses for IP for optometrists will rest with the General Optical Council (GOC). Optometrists who pass the final assessment will receive an endorsement on their GOC registration to denote the additional qualification.

If the legislative timetable proceeds as anticipated, it is likely that the first cohort of optometrists with the IP qualification will appear in 2009.

Supplementary prescribing

The Crown Report (1999) also recommended the implementation of dependent prescribing, which is now known as *supplementary prescribing*. The intention was to enable prescribing to specific health-care professionals for the management of long-term conditions. In 2003, further amendments were made to the Health and Social Care Act 2001 to enable supplementary prescribing by nurses and pharmacists who had completed specific supplementary prescribing training. Unlike IP there was no specific formulary, although unlicensed medicines and controlled drugs were initially restricted. The crucial aspect about supplementary prescribing is the specific legal requirement that there is an individual patient clinical management plan in place prior to supplementary prescribing. A medical or dental independent prescriber and the supplementary prescriber with the agreement of the patient must draw up the clinical management plan. The clinical management plan specifies the medical conditions, the range of medicines and the parameters for referral back to and review by the independent prescriber. The independent prescriber within this context is responsible for the initial assessment and diagnosis for the medical condition of the patient as outlined in the clinical management plan.

In 2005, Department of Health (DH) podiatrists, chiropodists, physiotherapists and radiographers became eligible to train and become supplementary prescribers (DH 2005). Restrictions in relation to controlled drugs and unlicensed medicines were lifted at the same time.

A consultation on IP of controlled drugs by nurse and pharmacist-independent prescribers (Consultation MLX 3338) to consider broadening the range of controlled drugs available to these groups of prescribers closed in July 2006. The outcome of this consultation is still awaited, although it is anticipated that the legislation will be laid before Parliament to lift the restrictions around the prescribing of controlled drugs for independent non-medical prescribers.

In July 2009 the Department of Health published a scoping report on a project that had focused on the evidence base to extend prescribing rights for groups of allied health professionals (DH 2009). The rationale for the project was to explore the impact on the quality of patient care of current prescribing arrangements for these professional groups. Based on the findings of a scoping exercise the following recommendations have been made to the chief professional officers within the Department of Health. There is a need to carry out a two-phase project to consider the following:

Phase 1

Further evidence to support the progression of

- physiotherapists and podiatrists to train as independent prescribers;
- dieticians to train as supplementary prescribers.

Phase 2

Further evidence to support the progression of

- radiographers to train as independent prescribers;
- speech and language therapists, orthoptists and occupational therapists to train as supplementary prescribers.

These are currently recommendations only so the timescale for any outcomes is as yet unknown.

The non-medical prescriber, however, has a duty of care to keep up to date with legal changes that apply to their own sphere of prescribing. Griffiths (2006) points out that before any practitioner prescribes or administers a drug he or she should ensure that they have the legal right to do so.

The National Prescribing Centre (NPC) issues daily current awareness bulletins http://www.npc.co.uk/ecab/ecab.htm, which non-medical prescribers and their employers can subscribe to in order to receive daily email alerts. The bulletins contain a wealth of information on health and social care and this includes updates on legal and safety aspects of medicines.

When prescribing medicines, the prescriber is judged against the standard of an experienced prescriber carrying out that role. McHale & Tingle (2007) have highlighted the unequivocal perspective that the DH (2006) has about this in that prescribers are accountable for every aspect of their decision making. This means that they should prescribe only those medicines that they know to be safe and effective and appropriate to the patient and the condition being treated.

It is also important to point out that laws that relate to consent, confidentiality and record keeping also apply to the non-medical prescribing role.

Professional standards as applied to non-medical prescribing

The NMC, Health Professions Council (HPC), The Royal Pharmaceutical Society for Great Britain (RPSGB) and DH work in partnership with the NHS strategic organisations and appropriate education providers in order to develop quality assurance arrangements for professional health-care education. This includes non-medical prescribing.

The Health Act 1999 determined the functions of the NMC, one of which is to determine the standards of education and training for admission to practise and give guidance about standards of conduct and performance.

The NMC was formerly referred to as the *United Kingdom Central Council for Nursing, Midwifery and Health Visiting*. The NMC (formerly UKCC) set specific standards for future professional practice known as *PREP* (1999). These were revised in April 2002 following the establishment of the NMC.

The rules to establish the new NMC register in August 2004 required that the time frames for meeting practice and CPD standards should both be 3 years. The date for implementation of this rule was August 2006 and has categorised into two domains, CPD education standard and practice standard. The requirements for the CPD standard is for registrants to undertake at least 35 hours of learning in 3 years prior to renewal of registration, maintain a personal profile of this learning activity and comply with requests from the NMC to audit compliance with these requirements.

The practice standard requires registrants to complete 450 hours every 3 years within the clinical area for which they hold professional registration.

The NMC is required by the Nursing and Midwifery Order 2001 (The Order) 'to establish from time to time standards of education, training, conduct and performance for nurses and midwives and to ensure the maintenance of those standards' [Article 3 (2)]. The Order also states 'the Council may make rules requiring registrants to undertake such continuing professional development, as it shall specify in standards'.

The NMC published *Standards of Proficiency for Nurse and Midwife Prescribers* in May 2006. This was to coincide with the implementation of the Independent Prescribing Regulations 2006 and set standards for the education and practice for all nurses and midwives who were either training or had qualified as prescribers. This includes community practitioner prescribers and independent and supplementary nurse prescribers. Standard 15 clearly states to the prescriber 'it is your responsibility to remain up to date with knowledge and skills to enable you to prescribe competently and safely'.

The NMC committed itself to developing the standards for CPD for nurse prescribers (Box 1.1) further, and interim measures were announced in September 2008 (NMC 2008a).

Box 1.1 Standards for CPD for non-medical prescribers registered with the NMC

- It is the non-medical prescriber's own accountability to remain competent and up to date with the tasks that are required within their prescribing role.
- Appraisal of CPD needs for non-medical prescribers should be part of an annual performance review using a recognised tool.

- This will determine the level of input for CPD for prescribers.
- Principles for CPD should equally apply to all levels of prescribers, for example, community practitioner nurse prescribers and non-medical prescribers.
- Applies to all prescribers irrespective of the clinical setting, for example, primary care, secondary care or private practice.
- A portfolio should be maintained in order to record achievement of learning needs and ongoing reflection.
- Employers should ensure that where CPD needs are recognised, they are supported by the employee and the employer and met to the satisfaction of all parties.
- Registrants are responsible for their own CPD but employers have a responsibility to help the registrants meet them.
- Practice requirements:
  - Should undertake assessments and make regular prescribing decisions
  - Does not apply to the number of prescriptions written
  - Hours spent in prescribing/making prescribing decisions should be counted.

The overall recommendations are to maintain the standards of PREP in that no additional time is required for either education or practice for CPD for non-medical prescribers. This could be viewed as a controversial move because the outcome of the Shipman Enquiry recommended mandatory CPD for all prescribers. The NMC, however, states that the Standards are considered to be an interim measure until the implementation of revalidation for all health-care professionals (DH 2007).

The rationale for standards of CPD for non-medical prescribers is in part due to the fact that one of the main categories of cases, which are reviewed by the NMC 'Fitness to Practice' panel, are in relation to medicines management issues, which includes prescribing.

The HPC have not published specific standards for CPD for non-medical prescribers but provide clear guidelines for CPD for all registrants (2006), which would apply where this concerns a non-medical prescribing role (Box 1.2).

Box 1.2 Standards for CPD for practitioners registered with the HPC

Maintenance of a continuous, up to date and accurate record of CPD to demonstrate that CPD activities

- are a mixture of learning activities relevant to current or future practice;
- seek to ensure that their CPD benefits the service user;
- present a written profile containing evidence of their CPD upon request.

All registered pharmacists have a professional obligation to maintain a record of their CPD. From autumn 2008, this is a mandatory requirement, and comprehensive guidance, templates and competencies have been drawn up to set standards and assist the practitioner with appropriate learning activities and frameworks for recording these. This includes additional competencies for independent and supplementary prescribing where this role is appropriate. The template is available at the website http://www.uptodate.org.uk/home/ PlanRecord.shtml.

Personal responsibility

All prescribers are liable to be responsible for their actions and accountable for keeping their skills and knowledge up to date, which is required in order to fulfil their prescribing role. This also involves consideration of the development of the ongoing scope of practice.

Hobden (2007) has suggested that prescribers should consider the use of the following tools to support CPD: 360 Appraisal, critical incident analysis, reflection and objective data, which may be available within practice.

All qualified non-medical prescribers are required to be assessed within a competency framework during prescribing training (NMC 2006).

Competency frameworks have potential as a useful tool when qualified as a prescriber in order to self-assess competency and identify CPD needs and integrate all of the tools as outlined by Hobden. This also supports the development of the portfolio, which is required to demonstrate CPD for non-medical prescribers. Ideally, a portfolio would demonstrate how, where and why the prescriber has achieved the relevant competencies and identify unmet learning needs.

The NPC Competency frameworks (NPC 2000, 2001, 2003a, 2004a, 2004b, 2006, 2007) are ideal for this and can be accessed at the website http://www.npc.co.uk/prescribers/competency_frameworks .htm.

An evaluation of independent nurse prescribing carried out by Latter *et al*. (2007) indicated that post-qualification, a high majority of participants had been able to maintain a wide range of the NPC competencies within their prescribing roles.

The competency frameworks also give the prescriber an opportunity to consider how they would like to receive CPD in relation to personal context and learning style (Figure 1.1). An example of how this could be adapted is illustrated below by using a sample of competencies.

Medicines management

In addition to guidance for non-medical prescribers the NMC (2008b) have also set standards for medicines management that covers aspects such as administration and storage of medicines. Similarly, the RPSGB

	I have had experience of doing this and can produce clear evidence	I have had experience of doing this but can produce no evidence to demonstrate this	I would like CPD on this topic in the following ways
Demonstrates the ability to use the British National Formulary safely by selecting the most appropriate drug, dose and formulation.	Reflection on prescribing case histories. Objective data, e.g. PACT		E-cab bulletins
Demonstrates the ability to identify inappropriate use of medications, including misuse, under and over-use.	Critical incident review		
Demonstrates the ability to review and report prescribing errors and near misses within a clinical governance framework.		I would like to explore this more fully within the context of my organisational setting	Action learning. Prescribing update study day

Figure 1.1 Use of a competency framework as a tool for CPD. PACT, Prescribing Analysis and Cost.

(2005) have set standards for the safe and secure handling of medicines from a team approach. The non-medical prescriber would be expected to have knowledge of these standards, especially where they are prescribing medicines that will be administered by other health-care professionals.

The role and responsibilities of the employer

The professional bodies (NMC, HPC & RPSGB) are clear that the employer has a responsibility to support non-medical prescribers in meeting their CPD needs.

In relation to non-medical prescribers who are registered with the NMC, employers are responsible for ensuring that the standards for PREP are met. Ideally this will be integrated into the non-medical prescribing policy (Chapter 3), which the employer will have put in place on behalf of the health-care organisation. The employer also has a duty to support the NMC Standards for CPD for non-medical prescribers (2008).

Scotland, Wales and Northern Ireland have devolved parliaments and have also developed legislation for non-medical prescribing. NHS Education for Scotland (NES) has a history of developing resources to support prescribers and their employing organisations. Accordingly the NES (2003) has developed a CPD tool to support the individual non-medical prescriber and identify the responsibility of the employer (Box 1.3). (http://www.nes.scot.nhs.uk).

Box 1.3 Employer's responsibility for CPD for non-medical prescribers (NES 2003)

- Identification of resources for CPD
- Use interprofessional opportunities for CPD
- Identify methods for CPD
- Identify appropriate timing and frequency of CPD
- Implement support systems for prescribers
- Record keeping and audit
  - What CPD has been undertaken within the organisation?
  - Have identified where CPD needs been met?
  - How have they been evaluated by participants?
  - What quality assurance processes are in place?
  - What are the outcomes of non-medical prescribing within practice?

This is a useful tool for all employers of non-medical prescribers. The individual chapters of this book provide a range of approaches and resources for CPD.

The NPC (2008) has recently published a guide for all NHS managers about what they need to know in relation to prescribing, the drugs bill and medicines management (http://www.npc.co.uk/policy/publications/publications.htm?type=all). This is a very useful resource for employers in order to support the CPD of prescribers because it contains basic facts about medicines, especially the legal framework and how medicines are supplied to patients and who should have the legal right to prescribe.

Accountability of the prescriber to the employer

The contract of employment outlines the instructions of the employer and it is anticipated that the employee will follow these instructions with appropriate levels of care and skill. If there is evidence of negligence, then the employer has the right to exert disciplinary powers. It is therefore important that the employment contract and job description of a non-medical prescriber outlines the boundaries of the prescribing role that the employer wishes the non-medical prescriber to hold. (Refer Section 1:2 of Appendix 1 for an exemplar job description, which includes non-medical prescribing.) Similarly, processes need to be in place to ensure that the non-medical prescriber can remain competent within that role and the employer has a duty to develop and uphold these.

In our experience of running non-medical prescribing courses and CPD updates, non-medical prescribers report that they are much clearer about their own professional boundaries once they have completed a prescribing course and have more confidence in negotiating the boundaries of their individual prescribing role with their employers and other health-care professionals within their multidisciplinary teams.

Test your knowledge about the law as it applies to non-medical prescribing

(See Section 1:3 of Appendix 1 for answers.)

Test your knowledge

1. What does professional responsibility mean in relation to non-medical prescribing?
2. What is the main legislation within the United Kingdom that relates to medicines?
3. What does this legislation regulate?
4. Name three resources, which can support a non-medical prescriber in keeping up to date with this legislation.
5. When did the Nurse Prescribers' Independent Extended Formulary become defunct?
6. What standards did the NMC implement on the same date?
7. Which professional groups can legally train and qualify as supplementary prescribers?
8. Which professional groups can practice as independent prescribers?
9. Which organisation has developed competency frameworks in order to support the CPD and education of non-medical prescribers?

Conclusion

It is an important aspect of professional responsibility for non-medical prescribers to keep up to date with the legal and professional frameworks that regulate and govern their prescribing role and the tasks that they are required to carry out in relation to this.

Professional bodies leave no doubt to registrants that this is a personal responsibility; however, managers and employers also have a responsibility to support and develop this and also keep up to date with the developments within these frameworks and how they apply to the health-care organisation.

This chapter has outlined the current legal and professional frameworks that relate to non-medical prescribing and has identified accessible resources to support and facilitate this process. These resources will support both the non-medical prescriber and his or her employer to promote the ongoing development of non-medical prescribing, which is safe and effective.

Key learning points

- The 1968 Medicines Act and the 1971 Misuse of Drugs Act regulate the supply, storage and administration of medicines.
- Subsequent amendments to these acts and The Prescription by Nurses Act, 1992 have broadened the scope of professional groups who have prescribing rights.
- Professional standards for CPD, education and practice for these professional groups are being developed accordingly and include the following:
  - Requirements for PREP
  - NMC *Standards of Proficiency for Nurse and Midwife Prescribers* (2006)
  - NMC *Standards for CPD for Nurse and Midwife Prescribers* (2008a)
  - Standards for CPD for practitioners registered with the HPC (2006)
  - Standards for CPD for pharmacists RPSGB (2008)
  - *Standards for Medicines Management* (NMC 2008b)
- Explicit within these standards is the individual responsibility for the non-medical prescriber to keep up to date. This can be underpinned by the following:
  - Competency frameworks
  - Reflection on practice, identification of unmet learning needs and preference for how these can be met
- Explicit within these standards is the responsibility of managers and employers:
  - Identification of CPD needs
  - Identification of appropriate resources to meet these needs
  - Access to appropriate educational resources

Key resources in Section Three

- List of web resources for keeping up to date with legal and professional issues
- Example job description, demonstrating the clear incorporation of non-medical prescribing as a key element of the role
- Answers to 'Test your knowledge' quiz.

References

Department of Health (1989) *Report of the Advisory Group on Nurse Prescribing (Crown Report)*. London, Department of Health.

Department of Health (1999) *Report of the Review of Prescribing, Supply and Administration of Medicines (Crown Report)*. London, Department of Health.

Department of Health (2005) *Supplementary Prescribing by Nurses, Pharmacists, Chiropodists/Podiatrists, Physiotherapists and Radiographers within the NHS in England: A Guide for Implementation*. London, Department of Health.

Department of Health (2006) *Medicine Matters: A Guide to Mechanisms for the Prescribing, Supply and Administration of Medicines*. London, Department of Health.

Department of Health (2007) *Trust, Assurance & Safety: The Regulation of Health Professionals in the 21st Century*. London, Department of Health.

Department of Health (2009) *Allied Health Professions Prescribing and Medicines Supply Mechanisms Scoping Project Report*. London, Department of Health.

Dimond, B. (2008) *Legal Aspects of Nursing*, 5th edition. Edinburgh, Pearson.

Griffiths, R. (2006) Legal requirements for prescribing, supply and administration of medicines. *Nurse Prescribing* 4(9): 365–370.

Health Professionals Council (2006) *Your Guide to our Standards for Continuing Professional Development*. London, HPC.

Hobden, A. (2007) Continuing professional development for nurse prescribers. *Nurse Prescribing* 5(4): 153–155.

Latter, S., Maben, J., Myall, M., Young, A. and Baileff, A. (2007) Evaluating prescribing competencies and standards used in nurse independent prescribers' prescribing consultations: An observation study of practice in England. *Journal of Research in Nursing* 12(1): 7–26.

McHale, J. and Tingle, J. (2007) *Law and Nursing*, 3rd edition. London, Butterworth-Heinemann.

NHS Education for Scotland (2003) *A Template for Continuing Professional Development in Prescribing*. Scotland, NES.

National Prescribing Centre (2000) *Competencies for Pharmacists Working in Primary Care*. Liverpool, NPC.

National Prescribing Centre (2001) *Maintaining Competency in Prescribing-an Outline Framework to Help Nurse Prescribers*. Liverpool, NPC.

National Prescribing Centre (2003a) *Maintaining Competency in Prescribing-an Outline Framework to Help Nurse Supplementary Prescribers*. Liverpool, NPC.

National Prescribing Centre (2004a) *Competency Framework for Prescribing Optometrists*. Liverpool, NPC.

National Prescribing Centre (2004b) *Maintaining Competency in Prescribing-an Outline Framework to Help Allied Health Professional Supplementary Prescribers*. Liverpool, NPC.

National Prescribing Centre (2006) *Maintaining Competency in Prescribing-an Outline Framework to Help Pharmacist Prescribers*, 2nd edition. Liverpool, NPC.

National Prescribing Centre (2007) *A Competency Framework for Shared Decision-Making with Patients: Achieving Concordance for Taking Medicines.* Liverpool, NPC.

National Prescribing Centre (2008) *What You Need to Know about Prescribing, The Drugs Bill and Medicines Management.* Liverpool, NPC.

Nursing and Midwifery Council (2006) *Standards of Proficiency for Nurse & Midwife Prescribers.* London, NMC.

Nursing and Midwifery Council (2008a) *Guidance for Continuing Professional Development for Nurse and Midwife Prescribers.* London, NMC .

Nursing and Midwifery Council (2008b) *Standards for Medicines Management.* London, NMC.

RPSGB (2005) *Code of Ethics.* London, The Royal Pharmaceutical Society of Great Britain.

RPGSB (2008) *Professional standards and Guidance for Continuing Professional Development.* London, Royal Pharmaceutical Society for Great Britain.

2 Prescribing Practice from the Employer's Perspective: The Rationale for CPD within Non-Medical Prescribing

Anne Smith and Sanjay Desai

Introduction

Making continuing professional development (CPD) available for practising independent prescribers has been challenging for all parties
involved. Whilst it is in the best interests of the employer to ensure
that practitioners remain updated and practice from a strong evidence
base, there is tension between who should be responsible for, and
who should finance, ongoing professional development. This chapter
explores some of the mechanisms adopted by Trusts to support practitioners to maintain some currency of knowledge in this important area.
It will also consider the individual's responsibility to remain updated
and briefly consider resources they could refer to, in order to maintain
and further develop their skills.

The organisational importance of continuing professional development

The Department of Health (DH 2002) acknowledges the importance of
lifelong learning amongst NHS staff as a key component of maintaining
a quality service, endorsing this view in various documents where they
offer guidance concerning post-qualifying professional education and
updating. Specifically, in 2004 the Department of Health published
a document that related to the CPD requirements of non-medical
prescribers (DH 2004). This is echoed in the governance agenda that

clearly stresses the need to promote CPD. Each NHS post has been mapped against its roles and functions in relation to representing organisational needs, defined in the Knowledge and Skills Framework. Personal development planning emphasises the developmental and CPD needs of the individual to fulfil their role. A cycle that incorporates outcomes related to personal development planning also follows the elements of the CPD cycle, these being reflection, planning, action and evaluation (NHS London Pharmacy Education and Training). Practitioners must accept some responsibility for their own professional updating and there are a variety of resources and tools available to do this. The Internet has enabled individuals to access a wide range of information and to network extensively, opening up channels of communication with all its attendant opportunities (Smith 2004).

Continuing education and continuing professional development

Clinicians need to understand the difference between continuing education and CPD. Attendance at a training event will constitute continued education but non-medical prescribers will need to reflect on what they have learned and how this will change their practice, which is activity that more closely reflects CPD (Hancox 2002). Simply being in attendance at events or conferences can be a passive activity and is insufficient to fully internalise the learning that has been achieved. Reflecting on and potentially changing practice or disseminating new knowledge as a result of these events demonstrates a critical approach and active engagement, thereby equating with a more dynamic approach to practice and personal development.

The manager's obligation to provide continuing professional development

Managers are presented with competing priorities and in a challenging financial climate, the budget for education is the first to be trimmed when economies are required to be made. As Tinson (2007) suggests, CPD for prescribing practitioners should be framed within a much greater infrastructure of professional development that is geared to upskilling individuals to meet workforce demands. It is therefore not an isolated provision. As Tinson comments, when independent prescribing was initially introduced, there were centrally led targets set regarding the number of practitioners to be trained. This inevitably led to managers focusing on achieving targets and perhaps not always considering whether training was linked to identified service need or indeed service enhancement. Draper and Clark (2007) discuss the type of CPD being commissioned by health-care organisations. Some Primary Care Trusts (PCTs) are addressing their responsibilities by providing 'quick-fix' in-house training rather than investing in more structured educational programmes. This satisfies their obligation to provide some form of CPD (NMC 2008a, 2008b) and may also be a means of tailoring education to their own organisational or local requirements. Without clear evidence, however, that more in-depth structured education enhances care, 'quick-fix' training approaches might meet an immediate obligation but tend to be less conducive to the lifelong learning agenda visualised by the Department of Health. This is a problem for training and education leads in Trusts who are trying to be creative in providing education to develop staff more broadly, in order to encourage practitioners to become critical thinkers as well as to develop and maintain their clinical expertise. It is vitally important to create a learning culture that permeates through the organisation so that CPD becomes an activity that is valued and sustained by practitioners themselves.

Identifying and meeting local learning needs

A major issue for PCTs is that the number of non-medical prescribers remains a small proportion of the number of clinicians across the Trust who require some form of CPD. This is further compounded by the fact that they come from a variety of areas of clinical practice and so the needs of individual practitioners will differ. Therefore, it would not necessarily be appropriate to run generic sessions for all non-medical prescribers, yet it would be costly to run courses in specific clinical specialties as there would be limited impact. Latter and Courtenay (2004) undertook a literature review examining the perceptions of independent nurse prescribing by district nurses and health visitors. Although their publications mainly report on the early days of nurse prescribing when the qualification was limited to these two professional groups, their findings in relation to their continued learning needs reflect the same issues that continue to be reported in more recent studies (Latter et al. 2007; Pontin & Jones 2007). Lessons can be learned from the findings reported as they are issues that continue to tax employers. For example, prescribers who were able to identify their CPD needs once they qualified included the necessity to consolidate their knowledge, particularly in relation to pharmacology, and the need to develop confidence in prescribing. They identified that informal support from team members was essential to developing their confidence and their practice. Having a 'buddy' or mentor in the practice setting to support them when newly qualified was also a suggestion. Many had been prescribing 'by proxy' for years, recommending treatments for general practitioners (GPs) to prescribe, but actually achieving the autonomy to write the prescription made them more nervous as they were responsible for making the final decision and signing the prescription (Otoway 2002).

Professional guidance

Since legislation was passed in 2006 that enabled nurses and pharmacists to prescribe extensively from the whole of the British National Formulary (DH 2006), it has been even more important for the regulatory bodies to demonstrate that systems are in place to protect the public. Therefore, whilst the initial training programmes are detailed, explicit and well monitored by the relevant authorities (Latter *et al.* 2007) there is less emphasis on monitoring of the CPD activity that non-medical prescribers are undertaking in order to maintain their knowledge and skills. Many nurses in particular, were trained as independent prescribers prior to the more recent legislative changes (DH 2006) and may not have been formally educated about these changes.

In the Nursing and Midwifery Council's publication on *Standards of Proficiency for Nurse Prescribers* (NMC 2006), there is explicit reference to CPD. Guidance to employers in relation to Practice Standard 15 states that employers have a responsibility to ensure that qualified prescribers have access to relevant CPD in order to maintain their competence. This has been re-enforced by a more recent circular from the NMC (2008a, 2008b) specifically relating to CPD for nurse and midwife prescribers, which advises that CPD activity in relation to independent and/or supplementary prescribing should be linked to practitioners' appraisals. Employers are vicariously liable for the actions of their staff and so have a vested interest in ensuring that they are safe and effective in their roles.

The first nurse independent prescribers were the V100 prescribers who were trained to prescribe from the Nurse Prescribers' Formulary. This qualification has now been revised and extended by the NMC (2006) to also incorporate the V150. Registered nurses working in the community are able to access training to enable them to prescribe from the limited formulary, now referred to as the *Nurse Prescribers' Formulary for Community Practitioners* (BMA, RPSGP 2007), which previously only permitted qualified community specialist practitioners to prescribe from the limited list of items. However, the principles associated with this type of prescribing are the same as with the V300 qualification, in that practitioners must be able to assess and diagnose their patients and prescribe safely and effectively. They are also required to develop the same skills in prescription writing, to understand the associated principles including pharmacokinetics, cost analysis and other related issues. It is imperative that employers are conscious that these practitioners should also have the opportunity to maintain their skills. If they are not regularly prescribing, then it is essential that they receive support in order to do so. It is known that many of those trained do not exercise their right to prescribe, preferring to adopt other mechanisms for administration or supply of medication. A variety of reasons for this are speculated upon by Otway (2002). Trusts find this a real challenge and are acknowledging this through appraisals and personal development plans. In some areas, Trusts are organising refresher training and support in order to give these nurses the confidence to re-commence and continue prescribing. However, in other areas, anecdotal evidence suggests that it seems likely that some of the original community practitioner/health visitor prescribers who do not use their prescribing qualification or update their skills face the possibility of their employers no longer permitting them to prescribe within their current role.

Registered nurses are accountable for their practice according to their *Code of Conduct* (NMC 2008c), as are pharmacists and allied health professionals, and must work within legal and ethical frameworks associated with professional practice. Therefore, they must ensure that they act always in the best interest of the patient and do no harm. Legally, individual practitioners are responsible for their actions to the public, to their employer and to their professional body and should be able to robustly defend their actions in the event of any problems occurring (Beauchamp & Childress 2001).

Organisational responsibility – the role of the Trust's non-medical prescribing lead

Trusts have a responsibility to provide appropriate support mechanisms for all prescribers to maintain their competence. Peer support such as forums or action learning sets are popular (NPC 2005) although attendance is sometimes difficult because of competing priorities. However, developing a strong culture of supervision and support amongst peers enables a group to take responsibility for their ongoing learning. This is a sound strategy from the point of view of the employer. Most Trusts have an identified non-medical prescribing lead. However, their role within the organisation is specified by each individual employer dependent on what the Trust priorities are. The role will also differ between primary and secondary care organisations. As the non-medical prescribing lead is often pivotal in driving forward the agenda and organising access to CPD and to CPD sessions, additional role(s) held by the non-medical prescribing lead therefore dictate the amount and type of training that is provided and there is no specified national standard. If, however, the practitioners themselves are pro-active and prepared to take ownership of their learning, together with a good steer from the Trust, they will be motivated to work in partnership for the benefit of all, and in particular, the client.

Latter *et al.* (2007) conducted the first national survey of nurse prescribers in which 62% of respondents reported that they were receiving some form of support or supervision, mostly sought from colleagues and peers informally. Of the respondents, 95% acknowledged that they kept up to date by personally accessing journals or through other private study. This study did have limitations associated with the respondents and the timing of the research. The method of data collection was a self-report questionnaire mainly targeted at senior nurses who had established a good working relationship with the doctors and were well supported in their role. They were also fairly newly qualified so their knowledge base was current, having only recently finished the formal taught component of the course. However, the authors conclude that although this group were recently qualified and so considered that their knowledge remained current employers should examine the local infrastructure for providing opportunities to maintain and update prescribers' knowledge. The implications of the study do highlight that there is a lack of an agreed national standard for the provision of CPD, and that access to CPD will therefore vary significantly from one organisation to another.

Meeting organisational and individual needs for CPD

Ultimately, for an accountable professional practitioner, CPD is an individual responsibility. It is also an activity that some individuals find difficult to manage when they are juggling the competing pressures of life and work. Many organisations provide 'in-house' courses and study days where the agenda is set in response to the suggestions of practitioners. More formal sessions can also be arranged locally, focussing on particular areas of expertise and organising guest speakers. Hancox (2002) however, advises that merely providing the opportunity to update does not necessarily mean that it has any benefit. Practitioners must be able to identify how to integrate learning within their practice to truly internalise the learning, and this, as highlighted earlier, suggests a clear difference between continuing education and CPD.

Gould *et al.* (2007) commented in a similar way that CPD was not always helpful either because it was delivered in too academic a format or at a level beyond the comprehension of attendees, although an alternative view expressed was that study days were too basic and therefore did not meet the needs of more senior staff. However, these findings do support the organisational observation that there are extremes of need in the provision of CPD at an organisational level and whilst there are clear areas or subjects of common interest, what might be useful to one professional group of non-medical prescribers will be unhelpful for another.

Identifying opportunities for CPD

Events can often be funded with the assistance of drug companies. This, however, can also pose a problem because of the fact that some drug representatives view non-medical prescribers as targets for aggressive marketing. Many Trusts have issued edicts to their non-medical prescribers concerning the influence of pharmaceutical company representatives and in some cases have issued protocols regarding acceptable behaviour or positively denied access. However, due to the cash-limited education budgets, many Trusts are now exploring opportunities to work in partnership with these groups in order to help meet the training needs of their employees. The Association of British Pharmaceutical Industry (ABPI) revised their Code of Practice on the 1 July 2008. Many of the changes are related to sponsorship declarations and now these must accurately reflect the nature of the company's involvement. There is also more guidance on hospitality and meetings. In addition, in May 08, the ABPI and the Department of Health published a toolkit to encourage joint working between the NHS and the pharmaceutical industry (DH/ABPI 2008).

Opportunities may be available to attend local or national conferences although the cost of these can be prohibitive. However, it is sometimes through attending such events that clinicians can find valuable opportunities to reflect on their own practice, hear the views of expert speakers and through such exposure can examine the very latest in developments and emerging ideas. There is merit in being encouraged to attend study days and conferences but equally those released to attend should then disseminate the knowledge through more local forums. Employers should maximise the benefits of any financial commitment made by recommending that prescribers who apply to attend these events must then in return be prepared to share the learning, thus feeding the investment back in to the organisation for the benefit of other prescribers.

Audit and analysis of prescribing habits could provide a method of identifying CPD needs. For individuals, this will provide a useful method of benchmarking practice, assessing whether prescribing is in line with their peers as well as in line with national trends. Primary Care prescribing is easily analysed via electronic Prescribing Analysis and Cost (PACT) data although this may not be as easily accessible in the acute sector where prescribing activity is more difficult to monitor. In primary care, local pharmacy representatives employed by Trusts to monitor prescribing patterns can offer useful advice regarding product costs and potential alternatives, as well as reinforcing any Trust protocols or prescribing formularies. Audit in relation to the clinical governance issues surrounding prescribing is, in addition, key to demonstrating safety and efficacy of non-medical prescribing practice. An example of an audit tool is incorporated in Section Three as a key resource (see Section Three, Appendix 2:2).

Monitoring CPD as part of appraisal

All these activities are integral to the appraisal process (Box 2.1). Each individual should view their appraisal as a vehicle for mapping their personal development needs and for highlighting how these could be effectively met. Importantly, through the appraisal process it is important to convey joint responsibility for CPD that whilst the organisation should provide access to CPD, it is the responsibility of the individuals to ensure their CPD is focused and relevant to their prescribing practice. The use of a framework to guide practitioners to consider those activities that their CPD involves may be useful (Figure 2.1). There are so many opportunities for practitioners to

Box 2.1　Examples of approaches to CPD

- Short update sessions
- Informal multidisciplinary meetings
- Audit
- Protected time for professional reading
- Performance appraisal
- Organised prescribing courses
- Critical incident analysis
- Clinical visits to other professionals involved in prescribing
- Mentoring/coaching
- Electronic updates
- Professional journals
- Clinical supervision
- Published articles
- Conference presentations
- Peer review.

Do you….	Do you comply with the listed activities? Yes/Some/No	How do you currently do this?	Do you think this method is satisfactory or would you prefer to do this differently? If so, how?
Reflect on your clinical decision making in relation to prescribing practice?			
Evaluate your consultation style with patients/clients in potential prescribing situations?			
Review and monitor your own practice as a prescriber in connection with professional and policy guidelines?			
Review and monitor your standard of prescription writing and record keeping?			

Figure 2.1 Example of an assessment tool for continuing professional development needs in prescribing.

Demonstrate knowledge of patient confidentiality in light of current legislation regarding the handling of personal data?					
Discuss prescribing issues with other professional prescribers?					
Access literature and data about prescribing?					
Demonstrate accountability with any links within the pharmaceutical industry?					
Work with members of the multi-disciplinary team in relation to prescribing?					
Reflect on your own prescribing practice, recognising your limitations, and identify when support from other prescribers is required?					
Provide support and guidance to other prescribers?					

Figure 2.1 *(continued)*

extend their knowledge so they should always be aware of 'serendipity learning'. Every opportunity for informal learning should be grasped whether it is some nugget of information seen in a journal or debating a critical incident and, importantly, acknowledged as a learning opportunity. Reflection is a powerful tool for examining actions. It can be undertaken alone or within a group but it is more beneficial if it is structured with clear outcomes to guide future practice. Often, it is a central component of educational courses (Smith & Jack 2005) but a poorly maintained discipline once a course is completed. However, it can be a precursor to research activity or the initiation of a change in practice. Historically, nurses have argued that they do reflect on their practice but that they do this opportunistically and informally and this information and learning from experience is not captured or recorded. In order for nursing to be acknowledged as a 'profession', it is essential for the body of nursing knowledge to be extended and developed. Research activity is pivotal to taking this forward, and reflective practice is often the first step. In the pressurised environment that characterises most workplaces, there is little time to stand back and consider any personal responsibility for this, considering it rather the domain of the academics in their ivory tower, but this is not the case as the most pragmatic and dynamic research is often that which is undertaken by the practitioner.

Maintaining the service

From the organisational perspective, there are wide implications for employers in managing the developmental needs of staff with regard to maintaining the service and finding the funding for practitioners to attend courses (Banning & Stafford 2007). Even if there is funding for staff to be released from their clinical or other responsibilities to attend CPD events or courses, actually identifying replacement staff is not easy. Non-medical prescribers are clinical specialist and senior personnel with their own caseload and finding appropriately qualified practitioners to undertake their duties may not be possible. Maintaining a service can therefore be a significant hurdle to overcome, together with parity of access to attend for all non-medical prescribers. Pragmatic issues such as these must be considered, whilst nurturing and encouraging CPD activity should be a priority for non-medical prescribing leads within the Trust. Managing these competing demands, supporting CPD activity for non-medical prescribers and maintaining the demands of an increasingly complex service truly relies on having an organisational culture of learning.

This echoes the sentiments of Senge (1990), who describes the characteristics of the learning organisation as being

'organizations where people continually expand their capacity to create the results they truly desire, where new and expansive patterns of thinking are nurtured, where collective aspiration is set free, and where people are continually learning to see the whole together.'

(Senge 1990; p. 3)

It corresponds with the governance philosophy of the 'no-blame culture' that should operate in Trusts (van Zwanenberg 2001) valuing openness and honesty regarding incidents and 'near misses', encouraging practitioners to view these as learning opportunities. Senge (1990) advocates that everyone has the capacity to learn but it is the culture within the workplace that either encourages or prevents the employees from taking the opportunities that are presented. Such activities as reflection and supervision are the catalysts for this and if the practitioners feel supported and valued, rather than threatened and demoralised, they will more readily explore potential or actual critical incidents and learn from them. Therefore, an organisation that is comprised of individuals who are continually open to discovery and new ideas will move forward effectively as the individuals and, so ultimately, the workforce are in a continual state of learning.

Conclusion

Evidence suggests that it is essential to have a systematic and joined up approach to CPD within Trusts for non-medical prescribers. Their role and expertise are pivotal to service re-design and enhancement, so investing in a structured approach will pay dividends. Latter *et al.*'s (2007) study indicated that practitioners are generally motivated to explore informal methods of maintaining their knowledge and skills by reading journals and working with colleagues to develop their roles. This reflects the findings of a survey by the National Prescribing Centre (NPC) in 2005, in which practitioners were asked in what ways the NPC could best support them in their role. The response indicated that there was a particular demand for providing information and exercises to enable them to maintain CPD. Latter *et al.'s* (2007) study had reported that 95% of the sample was engaging in such activities. In comparison, only half had received formal updating. Prescribers recognise that the most effective CPD is that which focuses educational updating towards addressing personally defined learning needs. It is about answering the burning questions that are relevant in the 'here and now'. These needs may change as non-medical prescribers meet different challenges in day to-day-practice. A recent example has been publicity about the legal implications of prescribing a mixture of medication for syringe-drivers (RCN, NCPC 2008). Once medication is mixed in a syringe-driver, it is essentially unlicensed. Raising awareness of such issues amongst practitioners is important and there should be access provided to a local forum for discussion. A further potential approach is a recommendation that arose from Otway's (2002) study that there is merit in publishing a local newsletter to provide some communication between local practitioners. It may be that such a publication is already being produced locally and that a corner could be incorporated specifically for prescribers to exchange views. A web-based forum is another option for providing a cheap and accessible way for prescribers to network when they may not be able to attend meetings. There are a variety of innovations that could be used but ultimately non-medical prescribers themselves must feel motivated to subscribe to and sustain such initiatives. Perhaps the best intervention to provide CPD is to foster the development of a learning organisation and to adopt a 'bottom up' approach, and give practitioners control of the agenda with the Trust educational and/or prescribing leads offering enthusiasm and appropriate support to sustain developments.

Key learning points

- CPD is everybody's responsibility.
- Practitioners must ensure that their knowledge is current and their practice evidence-based.
- Employers must provide appropriate opportunities for their staff to maintain their skills through relevant CPD activity.
- The organisational culture should promote all opportunities for learning both informally and formally.

Key resources in Section Three

- Useful websites
- Example of a clinical governance self-assessment tool for a health-care organisation to evaluate non-medical prescribing.

References

Banning, M. and Stafford, M. (2007) A hermeneutic phenomenological study of community nurses' CPD. *British Journal of Community Nursing* 13(4): 178–182.
Beauchamp, T. and Childress, J. (2001) *Principles of Biomedical Ethics*. 5th edition. New York, OUP.

British Medical Association, Royal Pharmaceutical Society of Great Britain, in association with Community Practitioners' Association and Royal College of Nursing (2007) *Nurse Prescribers' Formulary for Community Practitioners.* London, BMJ RPSGB.

Department of Health (DH) (2002) *Funding Learning and Development for the Healthcare Workforce.* London, Department of Health.

Department of Health (DH) (2004) *Extending Independent Nurse Prescribing within the NHS in England: A Guide for Implementation.* 2nd edition, London, Department of Health, http://www.dh.gov.uk/en/ Publicationsandstatistics/Publications/PublicationsPolicyAndGuidance/ DH_4006775 [Accessed 26 September 2008].

Department of Health (DH) (2006) *Improving Patients Access to Medicines: A Guide to Implementing Nurse and Pharmacist Independent Prescribing within the NHS in England.* London, Department of Health.

Department of Health (DH)/Association of British Pharmaceutical Industries (ABPI) (2008) *Moving beyond Sponsorship: Interactive Toolkit for Joint Working between the NHS and the Pharmaceutical Industry,* http:// www.dh.gov.uk/en/Publicationsandstatistics/Publications/ PublicationsPolicyAndGuidance/DH_082840 [Accessed 28 February 2009].

Draper, J. and Clark, L. (2007) Impact of professional education on practice. The rhetoric and the reality. *Nurse Education Today* 27(7): 515–517.

Gould, D., Drey, N. and Berridge, E. (2007) Nurses' experiences of continuous professional development. *Nurse Education Today* 27: 602–609.

Hancox, D. (2002) Making the move from continuing education to continuous professional development. *The Pharmaceutical Journal* 268(7180): 26–27.

Latter, S. and Courtenay, M. (2004) Effectiveness of nurse prescribing: a literature review. *Journal of Clinical Nursing* 13(1): 26–32.

Latter, S., Maben, J., Myall, M. and Young, A. (2007) Evaluating nurse prescribers' education and continuing professional development for independent prescribing practice. Findings from a national survey in England. *Nurse Education Today* 27(7): 685–696.

National Prescribing Centre (2005) *Results of surveying non-medical prescribers,* http://www.npc.co.uk/non_medical/Survey_Results_2005.pdf [Accessed 13 October 2008].

Nursing and Midwifery Council (NMC) (2006) *Standards of Proficiency for Nurse and Midwife Prescribers.* London, Nursing and Midwifery Council.

NMC (2008a) *Guidance for Continuing Professional Development for Nurse and Midwife Prescribers.* London, Nursing and Midwifery Council, http://www.nmc-uk.org/aFrameDisplay.aspx?DocumentID=4488.

NMC (2008b) *The PREP (Post-registration Education and Practice) Handbook.* London, Nursing and Midwifery Council, http://www.nmc-uk.org/ aFrameDisplay.aspx?DocumentID=4340.

NMC (2008c) *The Code. Standards of Conduct, Performance and Ethics for Nurses and Midwives.* London, Nursing and Midwifery Council.

Otway, C. (2002) The development needs of nurse prescribers. *Nursing Standard* 16(18): 33–38.

Pontin, D. and Jones, S. (2007) Children's nurses and nurse prescribing: a case study identifying issues for developing training programmes in the UK. *Journal of Clinical Nursing* 16: 540–548.

Royal College of Nursing and National Council for Palliative Care (2008) *Position Statement for Independent Prescribers*. London, RCN NCPC.

Senge, P. (1990) *The Fifth Discipline. The Art and Practice of the Learning Organization*. London, Random House.

Smith, A. (2004) The use of the internet to support the education of nurse prescribers. *Nurse Prescribing* 2(2): 26–30.

Smith, A. and Jack, K. (2005) Reflection. A meaningful task for students? *Nursing Standard* 19(26): 33–37.

Tinson, S. (2007) Government targets: getting the best from non-medical prescribing. In Brookes D. and Smith A. (Eds) *Non-medical Prescribing in Healthcare Practice. A Toolkit for Students and Practitioners*. Basingstoke, Palgrave.

Van Zwanenberg, T. (2001) Clinical governance in primary care: from blind-eye to no-blame culture in one short leap? *British Journal of Clinical Governance* 6(2): 83–86.

Useful websites

National Prescribing Centre:
http://www.npc.co.uk/

NHS Education for Scotland:
http://www.nes.scot.nhs.uk/prescribing/index.html

NHS London Pharmacy Education and Training:
http://www.londonpharmacy.nhs.uk/educationandtrsaining/ksf/ksf.aspx

Nursing and Midwifery Council:
http://www.nmc-org.uk/

The Association of the British Pharmaceutical Industry:
http://www.abpi.org.uk/

3 Writing and Maintaining a Non-Medical Prescribing Policy for Your Organisation

Michael Fanning

Introduction

The advent of non-medical prescribing has introduced a new and exciting era for a whole range of health professionals and the act of prescribing has dramatically changed the dynamics of the health-care team. These changes can be seen in daily practice and experienced by patients who access services, with examples that range from the independent prescriber working in a minor injury unit to the consultant pharmacist working with complex care management pathways in cancer care.

Whilst each health professional will work within his or her professional scope of practice as set out by the appropriate regulator and guidance from professional associations, it is also an absolute necessity for the employing organisation to have a clear framework for non-medical prescribing.

This chapter discusses the areas which organisations should include in the development of a non-medical prescribing policy and, as an appendix to the chapter, sets out an illustrative example of a non-medical prescribing policy (see Section Three, Appendix 3:2), developed from a combination of policies taken from a variety of acute and primary care trusts that serves to illustrate those areas which can be included.

Background to clinical governance

Clinical governance was introduced as a concept in 1998 (DH 1998) as a framework to ensure that all National Health Service (NHS) organisations have proper processes for monitoring and improving quality of care. It brought together a number of methods for improving quality that were already in existence, namely, putting research into practice, collecting information to measure performance against standards, providing ongoing education for all health professionals and managing and learning from complaints (Scally & Donaldson 1998). Clinical governance clearly stresses the organisational accountability for developing and monitoring standards and a part of this process is the organisational requirement to develop local policies that enable professionals to guide and develop practice in specific areas. Importantly, clinical governance also puts the onus on the organisation to provide opportunities for continuing professional development (CPD).

Developing the policy

There is no single approach to the development of a policy, although the purposes of a non-medical prescribing policy are to set out what can be expected of the organisation, the prescribers within the organisation and where the responsibility for governance arrangements lies.

The aim of any policy is to provide a clear statement of intent and in the case of clinical practice the policy will also state very clearly the expected behaviour of practitioners in providing a particular treatment, therapy or service. It will need to include a clear statement of the organisational responsibilities in supporting non-medical prescribing. It is helpful in the introduction of the policy to provide a brief context relating to its need. For non-medical prescribing this should be written in a way that summarises the history and development of non-medical prescribing and provides a brief understanding, by explaining and differentiating between independent and supplementary prescribing, the professional and legal status of prescribers and the current perspective from both a professional and legal position. During recent years, there have been updates and amendments to the law relating to non-medical prescribing occurring at a frequent rate, and for this reason any policy should note any potential changes that may be subject to legislation or be influenced by a national inquiry, for example, Shipman. For the same reason, any policy requires very regular review, particularly, given the changing nature of professional developments and the introduction of professional guidance that relates to prescribing not only in law but also in guidance issued from time to time by professional bodies such as the Nursing and Midwifery Council (NMC), the Royal Pharmaceutical Society of Great Britain (RPSGB) and the Council for the registration of Allied Health Professionals (AHPs).

It is important to set the scene at the outset of the policy and not to make assumptions that all clinical staff will fully understand the non-medical prescribing agenda, and for managers at all levels to understand the implications of supporting practice through various stages, including the ongoing support of prescribers once qualified. The latter is clearly important in considering the arrangements within the organisation for CPD, the arrangements for which, with clear lines of responsibility, should be set out.

Administering and prescribing

There is still some confusion amongst health-care staff about the terminology used in the actual delivery of medicines to their patient. Regrettably, anecdotal accounts can still be described where nurses who are not eligible to prescribe will state that they have prescribed a medicine, when in fact, they mean administer. In addition, there are the situations where the same nurses may be able to supply and administer medicines under a Patient Group Direction (PGD) (HSC 2000/26) and there is a general miscomprehension that this equates to prescribing. It is important that there be a clear explanation about the differences to avoid confusion, not just amongst practitioners but also for the benefit of patients.

The supply and administration of medicines under a PGD will have advantages for certain patient groups and under particular circumstances. It must be remembered that the use of PGDs has to be for the advantage of the patient and, where improving service delivery to patients may mean access to a wider range of practitioners, which may not be possible under non-medical prescribing. This section must therefore clearly state that the PGD does not allow 'prescriptions to be written' to authorise another practitioner to administer medicines. A list of approved PGDs must be kept by the organisation and this is usually the responsibility of either the lead pharmacist or nurse for non-medical prescribing. Arrangements must also be made for the review and updating of PGDs together with audit on a regular basis.

Differences between types of prescribers, that is, supplementary and independent prescribers, should be described, particularly highlighting any limitation to the type of medicines that can be prescribed from the formulary (DH 2002, 2005). A brief explanation should also be provided about the clinical management plan (CMP). The use of the CMP needs to be understood in as much as it changes the dynamics of the traditional prescribing relationship and is a good example of patient engagement. This section of the policy may conclude by outlining examples of clinical care where practitioners are prescribing, for example, in a nurse-led rapid access chest pain clinic, chronic disease management or a pharmacist prescribing parenteral nutrition.

Strategic intent

This section should make reference to Department of Health Guidance (DH 2006). There should be a brief statement about the strategic intent of the organisation and an outline of the plan, which will be developed (Box 3.1). This should include the following:

Box 3.1 Strategic intent of a non-medical prescribing policy

- Recognition of the benefits to patients
- The initial range of clinical pathways where patients could benefit
- An acknowledgement that the development of non-medical prescribing needs to be service driven
- The need for prescribing to be included in business plans;the potential for service redesign to support the non-medical prescribing agenda
- Identification of support measures for staff and how transition will be maintained whilst staff extend their roles and the services they currently provide
- Methods of communication to inform patients and clinical and non-clinical staff
- Timescales for implementing non-medical prescribing
- The named lead director who will be responsible for the implementation plan.

Key principles of non-medical prescribing

The key principles that need to be discussed include the need to ensure that patient safety is not compromised, and the need to express that the implementation of non-medical prescribing must offer clear benefits for patients. There has to be agreement from the patient or, when appropriate, the carer or parent. Reference should also be made to the fact that non-medical prescribing should support multidisciplinary working and must also utilise the best knowledge and skills of practitioners. The appropriateness of PGDs should also be mentioned as also how these might continue to be the most appropriate approach to the administration of medicines in specific situations. Finally, there should be reference to the need to ensure that prescribing and dispensing responsibilities and ensuring that prescribing and administration should, where possible, be separate, to support the principle of patient safety and governance.

Framework for non-medical prescribing

The main body of the policy will need to describe the responsibilities of practitioners, as specified in Box 3.2.

Box 3.2 Framework for non-medical prescribing

Independent prescribing: This should include setting out the parameters of prescribing only for medical conditions that the practitioner is competent to treat, taking full accountability for his or her own prescribing.

Supplementary prescribing: This should include the partnership relationship between the independent and supplementary prescribers and the requirement for training (National Prescribing Centre (NPC) 2003; 2005). The policy should specify the need for a doctor or a dentist to undertake the independent prescriber role and their responsibility in determining which patients may benefit. The methods of communication between the two prescribers must be stated, together with how the CMP will be drawn up, monitored and reviewed. It is also necessary to include how responsibility for CMPs can be transferred from one independent prescriber to another. The discretion and variances of prescribing within the CMP will also need to be clearly stated.

Responsibilities of the independent medical prescriber and the supplementary prescriber: For the independent prescriber this needs to include the initial clinical assessment, formulation of the CMP, undertaking reviews and reporting adverse incidents following local organisational policies, through to national reporting mechanisms such as the National Patient Safety Agency and the Medicines and Healthcare Products Regulatory Agency. The supplementary prescriber is responsible for the management of the patient's condition in accordance with the CMP, including monitoring and assessment of the patient, working within their Code of Professional Conduct, referring to the independent prescriber if the agreed clinical reviews are not undertaken and ensuring that contemporaneous records are kept within the shared patient record.

Working together: This should include the need for both prescribers to work together and the recognition that both prescribers may work in more than one prescribing relationship.

Whilst the precise layout of the clinical management plan can vary according to organisational need, it must include the following information (Box 3.3):

Box 3.3 Content of the Clinical Management Plan

- Name of the patient
- Illness or conditions that may be treated by the supplementary prescriber
- The dates on which the plan is to take effect and to be reviewed
- Reference to the class or description of medicines or appliances, which can be prescribed or administered, including reference to published national or local guidelines, and stating when the dose, frequency and formulation can be varied
- Restrictions or limitations about the strength or dose of medicines

- Relevant warnings about known sensitivities of the patient or known difficulties of the patient with particular medicines or appliances
- Arrangements for the notification of suspected or known drug reactions, managing incidents which might lead to deterioration in the health of the patient, and making a referral to the independent prescriber.

Examples of templates can be found where there is shared and non-shared access to the CMP at http://www.cmponline.info and further examples of plans can be found using the site's search facility. A policy can additionally illustrate the use of CMPs within the organisation by providing examples. Arrangements for the review of CMPs must also be included together with how the plan will be ended. A useful tool to assist practitioners in developing shared decision making has been produced by the NPC (Clyne *et al.* 2007).

Professional requirements to become a non-medical prescriber

For all practitioners there are specific professional requirements to fulfil the appropriate regulatory body criteria, in order to become a non-medical prescriber. As well as identifying the national requirements, additional local requirements, such as a minimal amount of experience working at a particular level of expertise, inclusion of prescribing responsibilities in the job description, a contract being held by a sole employer and approval that all requirements have been met through an internal group who have responsibility for overseeing non-medical prescribing may be stated. Further guidance and up to date information about the status of practitioners' ability to prescribe nationally can be provided either by the RSPGB, NMC or the Health Professions Council and it is useful to provide contact details for these organisations within the policy.

Registering as a non-medical prescriber with the organisation

This section of the policy should provide clear direction for prescribers, whether newly qualified or those with experience transferring from one employer to another, about whom to contact within the organisation and any process that must be followed before starting to prescribe. A registration form produced by the organisation should be used and details should include job title, contact details, site(s) where prescribing will be undertaken, details of the non-medical prescribing course undertaken, evidence from the regulatory body on prescribing status, details of the clinical area and job description, as well as signatures of the prescriber and line manager. Specific local criteria may include the need for the employing manager and independent prescriber (for the supplementary prescriber) to be satisfied that the necessary skills and knowledge have been demonstrated. The requirement to check the status of the prescriber with the appropriate professional regulator must also be included, together with who will be responsible for this and how the status will be recorded within the organisation.

Local register

Details of a local register of non-medical prescribers should include where this can be accessed within the organisation and who will be responsible for its maintenance. Information should also be provided about the responsibility of the practitioner to maintain their local registration. For example, this may include advice relating to undertaking a period of supervised practice if the practitioner transfers from one speciality to another. Where practitioners have undergone a period of extended leave the practitioner should be required to undertake to work with a senior clinician to ensure that both confidence and competence to prescribe have been maintained, in addition to the requirement to maintain their individual CPD. The local register will also need to reflect any change of personal circumstances, such as change of name.

Prescribing what and for whom

A description outlining what may be prescribed and from which formulary should be included. These will range from General Sales List medicines to appliances and foods to Prescription-only Medicines (some of which may have restrictions). It is common practice to make sure medicines are also included in the local formulary of the organisation. Specific reference should also be made to the responsibilities of the supplementary prescriber and any restrictions placed by the organisation, for example, relating to the local formulary. Restrictions on prescribing for the individual need of the prescriber and the prescriber's family must be clearly stated, and this is supported by both national and local policy.

Documentation and associated prescribing paperwork

A clear statement of expectation must include the local prescribing paperwork to be maintained, particularly to support a good record of the medication history. Agreement for the designation of prescribers and the mark on drug charts and prescriptions will need to be stated, for example, 'PSP' means 'pharmacist supplementary prescriber'.

FP10 prescriptions

The use of FP10 prescriptions is controlled and the prescriber must follow local arrangements for their use. The example prescribing policy attached sets out one approach (see Section Three; Appendix 3 Page 163), although local practice varies, and the policy should reflect this. However, this may include seeking authorisation from the appropriate manager of services and the finance manager.

Record keeping

Guidance on the management of records according to local protocol should be included as well as general reference to the regulatory and professional bodies.

Administration of medicines against prescriptions

In keeping with the principles of patient safety and to comply with the principles of governance, advice should be given that where possible the item prescribed should be administered by another appropriately qualified health-care professional. Where this might compromise patient care and the prescriber administers the medicine, a statement should be made about the principles of following all safety checks to ensure that the right patient receives the right medicine, in the right dose by the right method of administration.

Dispensing

Prescriptions from non-medical prescribers should be dealt with in the same manner as those from medical prescribers. The process for pharmacy staff should include the checking of the name of the prescriber against the local register. Where appropriate schemes are in place, it is possible for nurses and midwives to supply an appropriate pre-packed and labelled medicine from the pharmacy against the prescription of the prescriber. Arrangements should be in place to ensure that medicines that have been prescribed by a pharmacist prescriber are not dispensed by the same prescriber.

Security and safe handling of prescriptions

Guidance on the handling of prescription forms, drug charts and FP10 prescriptions should be included and this should include suspected or actual loss. Where electronic prescribing is used the prescriber should be advised of the fundamentals of password protection.

Adverse drug reactions

Where a patient has an adverse reaction to a medicine, the prescriber must be advised to inform the patient's consultant and to ensure the incident is recorded in the patient record. In circumstances where there is an adverse incident or near miss, clear guidance needs to be given about the use of local incident reporting together with using the National Patient Safety Agency's national reporting system. Where appropriate, the adverse incident should be reported via the yellow card system to the Medicines and Healthcare Products Regulatory Agency. The prescriber should also be advised to record any incidents in their personal reflective log and identify potential learning needs.

Annual review

Arrangements should be included for the annual review of the CMP and patient care for patients under the care of supplementary prescribers unless more frequent reviews have already taken place.

Continuing professional development (CPD)

The organisation will need to ensure that all prescribers undertake their professional responsibility to participate in CPD and that training needs are included in personal development plans and linked to the appropriate knowledge and skills framework. Organisations should develop fora to support non-medical prescribing CPD activities and these should be made known to prescribers. It is important that the policy both reinforces and supports professional guidance with relation to CPD and it should of course be noted that an organisation does have the responsibility to make CPD available to a variety of web-base links to support CPD activity that can also be included (e.g. NPC (http://www.npc.co.uk), Pharmacy Post-graduate Education (http://www.cppe.man.ac.uk), Nursing and Midwifery Council (http://www.nmc-uk.org).

Associations with the pharmaceutical industry

Prescribers will need to be aware of the guidance from their own organisation and the DH on working with representatives from the pharmacy industry.

Liability

The responsibility of both the employer and the employee should be clearly stated as well as that both parties are responsible for ensuring the compliance of non-medial prescribers practising within approved policies and structures.

Professional indemnity

Whilst the employer will indemnify the practitioner who practices within the approved framework, it is advisable to include the suggestion that professional indemnity insurance is accessed either through membership of a professional organisation or through an insurance policy.

Clinical governance

Part of the assurance for satisfying clinical governance requirements will be the development of an overall policy that is approved according to local arrangements and frequently monitored and reviewed. A risk assessment and management plan should be included as a matter of best practice and an equality impact assessment undertaken to mitigate potential discrimination against patient groups. Matters often overlooked include making sure that version control (including amendments), review dates and authors by job role are included. Once approved, the policy should also have a detailed implementation plan devised to support the embedding of the policy in the organisation.

Patient information

Good quality patient information must be available to patients to explain the role of the prescriber, the benefit to the patient, assurances about practice and who to contact about potential concerns. It is useful to append examples of locally or nationally used educational materials as an appendix to the policy and to ensure that these are readily available within the organisation.

Selection of potential prescribers

A checklist should be produced and completed to assist the potential prescriber before applying for a programme. For the potential prescriber they must be able to provide assurance that they have the appropriate specialist knowledge and that they will be able to prescribe on completion of the programme, and they must also ensure that they have the support of their manager. It should be clear that the service they provide will support patients' needs through the ability to prescribe. It is incumbent on the organisation to be very clear regarding the selection of prescribers prior to putting individuals forward to train, according to requirements set out by the professional bodies, particularly the NMC. The manager must demonstrate an understanding of the implications for the service and that there is capacity to ensure that the potential pre-scriber will have support during their training. In addition, the manager will need to ensure that a robust clinical governance framework is in place and that there is access to a prescribing budget. The non-medical prescribing lead(s) for the organisation must be satisfied that patient safety will not be compromised, there is maximum benefit to patients and it is the best use of the practitioner's skills.

Monitoring practice

In addition to the activities associated with CPD and staff personal formal reviews, it is recommended that professional or line managers of prescribers undertake periodic reviews. The NMC in particular now suggests that discussion of CPD undertaken, as well as future needs, form part of an appraisal process in order that individual activity can be monitored. The types of issues reviewed can include the types of medicines being prescribed and how frequently, benefits to patients, problems implementing prescribing, the potential effect on colleagues in other organisations and use of a reflective log. This should assist where there is potential poor performance or a lack of confidence on the part of the prescriber, and a proactive approach can be taken to address issues.

Monitoring of non-medical prescribing practice can take place locally at a directorate or practice level, particularly in a large Trust, or at an organisational level, or indeed both. The policy should contain some detail as to how this will be undertaken, who will be responsible for conducting the audit, the approach(es) used to audit and how the outcomes of audit will be communicated to the organisation.

Organisational roles and responsibilities

This section will need to identify the role of committee(s) within the organisation that will have a specific role in supporting the devel-opment and introduction of non-medical prescribing. This may also include a requirement for the committee(s) to receive an annual report about the activity of non-medical prescribers. As previously mentioned there must be assurance around the governance arrangements and the governance committee will have a specific role to ensure that an approved framework is in place, which ensures that practices are within the law. Professional boards within the organisation will have a responsibility to ensure that the necessary framework supports the potential development of professional roles and services. The local forum, which has specific responsibility for non-medical prescribing and PGDs, will likely need to ensure the detailed work of ensuring that the policy is implemented, to check the policy against the governance framework, to liaise with other groups or committees, facilitate CPD activities and produce the annual report. The chief pharmacist will also need to ensure that the policy satisfies the overall requirements for medicines management. Managers responsible for services will need to plan for appropriate staff to be released for training.

Useful contacts

It is often helpful to include in the final section useful contact details within the organisation, the higher education institutes, health authority and websites.

Final section

The final section can include references to other local or national polices such as those for record keeping and handling of FP10 prescriptions. It may also be helpful to include a glossary of terms.

Conclusion

The development and agreement of an organisational policy fulfils the requirement for governance arrangements around non-medical prescribing, and provides a reference point for non-medical prescribers as well as their managers as to the organisational frameworks for implementation and monitoring practice. In addition, the policy offers clear explanations to those often-posed questions surrounding issues such as accountability, team working and process. The example policy (Page 163) serves only as an illustration of the points raised in this chapter and is developed from several policies drawn together from acute and primary care trusts.

Key learning points

- It is an absolute necessity for the employing organisation to have a clear framework for non-medical prescribing (NMP).
- The NMP framework will be at the heart of the clinical governance agenda for the organisation.
- The NMP framework should outline the necessity to the organisation of
  - PGDs;
  - administration of medicines;
  - independent prescribing;
  - supplementary prescribing.
- The NMP framework should outline the strategic intent of the NMP policy.
- The key principles of an NMP policy are as follows:
  - Professional requirements to become an NMP
  - The remit of prescribing roles within the organisation
  - Arrangements for record keeping
  - The use of appropriate prescription forms
  - Who can administer against an NMP prescription
  - Arrangements for dispensing NMP prescriptions
  - Security and handling of prescriptions
  - Annual review of CMPs
  - Arrangements for CPD
  - Relationships with the pharmaceutical industry
  - Liability
  - Professional indemnity.

Key resources in Section Three

- Useful websites
- An example of an organisational non-medical prescribing policy.

References

Clyne, W., Ganby, T. and Picton, C. (2007) *A Competency Framework for Shared Decision-Making with Patients*, 1st edition. Liverpool, Medicines Partnership Programme, National Prescribing Centre.

Department of Health (DH) (1998) *A First Class Service. Quality in the New NHS*. London, Department of Health.

Department of Health (DH) (2002) *Extending Independent Nurse Prescribing within the NHS in England*, 2004 2nd edition. London, Department of Health.

Department of Health (DH) (2005) *Supplementary Prescribing by Nurses, Pharmacists, Chiropodists/Podiatrists, Physiotherapists and Radiographers within the NHS in England - a Guide for Implementation*. London, Department of Health.

Department of Health (DH) (2006) *Improving Patients Access to Medicines: A Guide to Implementing Nurse and Pharmacist Independent Prescribing within the NHS in England*. London, Department of Health.

HSC (2000/26) *Patient Group Directions*. England, Department of Health.

National Prescribing Centre (2003, 2005) *Supplementary Prescribing – A Resource to Help Healthcare Professionals to Understand the Framework and Opportunities*. Liverpool, National Prescribing Centre.

Scally, G. and Donaldson, I. (1998) Clinical governance and the drive for quality in the new NHS in England. *British Medical Journal* 317: 61–65.

4 Organising CPD for Non-Medical Prescribers at a Regional Level

Fiona Peniston-Bird

Introduction

In this chapter, I will use my experiences both as a regional prescribing facilitator and an independent non-medical prescribing (NMP) consultant to provide examples of how to organise continuing professional development (CPD) for NMPs.

This cannot be explored without considering the structure of the National Health Service (NHS) and how national health-care policy is devolved to the regional level and how this has influenced the NMP agenda.

The chapter explains the current structure of strategic health authorities (SHAs), how this has changed over recent years and the implications for NMP. The following sections include working examples of networking and learning from a national prescribing forum and how these translate to organising CPD at a regional level. I will then discuss possibilities for motivating NHS Trust NMP leads at an organisational level to develop CPD frameworks such as developing a CPD business case, commissioning a training needs analysis and commissioning the provision of therapeutic workshops. I will also provide some practical application of ideas for running CPD prescribing workshops at a regional or local level.

This chapter is based on the perspective that in spite of many changes within the United Kingdom to extend prescribing rights to nurses and other groups of health-care professionals, there is a lack of standardisation in providing CPD for those groups who have undertaken NMP training.

The structure of the NHS within the United Kingdom

The National Health Service (NHS) was set-up in 1948 as part of the post-war welfare state reforms. It is one of the largest organisations in Europe and is recognised by the World Health Organisation as a world leading health service.

Within the United Kingdom, the NHS employs more than 1.5 million people. Of those, approximately half are professionally and clinically qualified. This includes 90,000 doctors, 35,000 general practitioners (GPs), 400,000 nurses and 16,000 ambulance staff.

The NHS services are funded from the central government via public taxation. NHS services in England, Northern Ireland, Scotland and Wales are managed separately. This is in line with the devolved parliaments, which results in some differences, especially in regard to legislation. This has had some implications for the development of NMP in that amendments to the law have not been implemented at the same time between the separate countries. Having said this, the NHS in these countries remains very similar and it is regarded as a single unified system.

In 2002, throughout the whole of England 28 SHAs were set up in order to deliver the *New Labour* health-care policy agenda, which were intended to improve health services at a local level by ensuring that local NHS organisations were working effectively. SHAs manage NHS locally and are a key link between the Department of Health and health-care organisations at the front of health-care delivery.

On 1 July 2006, the 28 SHAs were reduced to 10. However, they continue to have the same role in overseeing local health-care organisations, in particular health-care trusts. These include Primary Care Trusts (PCTs), acute health-care trusts (secondary care) and mental health-care trusts.

PCTs oversee health-care delivery within primary care and have a major role in commissioning local secondary health-care services with a control of approximately 80% of the NHS budget. As they are situated locally it is assumed that they are best positioned to understand the health-care needs of the local community and ensure that local health-care services are functioning effectively. PCTs support 29,000 GPs and 18,000 NHS dentists.

Secondary care trusts, which are sometimes better known as acute health-care trusts encompass hospital care, which provides emergency or elective care, planned specialist medical care or surgery following referral from primary care.

Mental health care trusts are also overseen by SHAs; mental health-care trusts provide mental health-care services to patients both in hospital and community settings.

Up until 2006/2007 when the NHS underwent significant structural changes, each of the 28 SHAs had an assigned regional NMP facilitator or lead role.

The national context for the development of non-medical prescribing

The NHS Plan (DH 2000) promoted changes in professional roles and boundaries in order to meet modern health-care demands and set out a 10-year plan for modernisation of the NHS. Related health-care policies, *National Service Framework for Mental Health* (DH 1999), *Supporting People with Long-Term Conditions* (DH 2005a) and *Creating a Patient-Led NHS Delivering the NHS Improvement Plan* (DH 2005b), emphasise the importance of multidisciplinary involvement in prescribing and medicines management. The national development of NMP roles have been influenced by these policies and NMP is a complex arena, which relates to many aspects of healthcare.

The NHS Plan (2000) outlined 10 key roles for nurses, one of which was the prescribing of drugs and medicines. This document also recommended extension of prescribing rights to other professional groups.

As an outcome of *The NHS Plan,* the DH (2002) set specific targets that 10,000 nurses to have qualified as extended independent or supplementary prescribers by the end of 2004. This was an ambitious projection and the then policy lead for NMP within the Department of Health made a suggestion to change the term of 'targets' to 'aspirations'.

A range of incremental policy directives and legislation followed, which now enables nurses and pharmacists who meet specific criteria to undertake training as independent and supplementary prescribers and for physiotherapists, chiropodists/podiatrists and radiographers who meet specific criteria to undertake training as supplementary prescribers.

The whole expansion of non-medical prescribing was a high priority for the Department of Health. *The NHS Improvement Plan, Putting People at the Heart of Public Services and Creating a Patient-led NHS* (DH 2004, 2005b) identifies that patients should have increased choice and access to a wider range of services; this includes increasing the range of health-care professionals who can prescribe drugs to patients. Patients should have flexible access to services shaped around individuals' needs and preferences, rather than, an expectation that people will fit the system.

Improving roles in a more flexible workforce is a further objective of the NHS Improvement Plan. NMP utilises the skills of the NHS workforce and improves access to medicines for the patient. It enables the patient to receive timely episodes of care by the most appropriate health-care professional.

Legislation within Scotland has mirrored the English developments of NMP. Rather than SHAs it was the NHS boards in Scotland that were tasked with developing a strategic plan for NMP to include independent prescribing by nurses and pharmacists. The NHS boards typically consisted of senior managers, doctors, nurses, pharmacists and local drug and therapeutic committees.

Where medicines legislation permits the introduction of supplementary and independent NMP in the United Kingdom, it is for England and the devolved administrations in Wales, Scotland and Northern Ireland to decide whether and how NMP is implemented.

In 2002, a policy decision was made in Wales not to introduce extended independent nurse prescribing in advance of supplementary prescribing. In October 2003, the NHS regulations (Wales) were amended in order to allow supplementary prescribing. The Welsh Assembly Government sponsored a total of 250 nurses and pharmacists to undertake training. In 2006, a task force group for the extension to independent prescribing for nurses and pharmacists was established in Wales. Independent prescribing for nurses and pharmacists in Wales came into effect on 1 February 2007.

In spite of all of these policy directives, in my experiences from being involved with NMP, the uptake for training has been relatively slow (Box 4.1).

Box 4.1 Numbers of non-medical prescribers in the United Kingdom

Department of Health Statistics for qualified non-medical prescribers January 2009 (Personal communication)	
Community Practitioner Formulary Nurse Prescribers	26,357
Nurse Independent Prescribers	13,705
Physiotherapist Supplementary Prescribers	109
Chiropodist/podiatrist Supplementary Prescribers	75
Radiographer Supplementary Prescribers	19
Pharmacist Independent Prescribers	855
Pharmacist Supplementary Prescribers	1478

The role of a regional non-medical prescribing facilitator

With a background in nursing and health visiting, I was one of the first nurses in the United Kingdom who undertook the Extended

Independent Nurse Prescribing training in early 2002. I subsequently set up and ran a minor ailments clinic within a GP practice in Shoreham, West Sussex.

I was frustrated by a lack of support, infrastructure and CPD for my prescribing role, and was therefore delighted to be appointed to the role of Non-Medical Prescribing Facilitator for the Strategic Health Authority (SHA) covering Surrey and Sussex in 2003.

The role of NMP facilitator was created by the Surrey and Sussex SHA to inspire, support and lead the development of NMP within health-care organisations across the region.

The project for the role of NMP facilitator was supported by a ring-fenced budget, which was allocated by the Department of Health. The Surrey and Sussex SHA aimed to support the strategic development of high quality NMP programmes, which were delivered by local higher educational institutions (HEIs).

The post of NMP facilitator required an ability to interpret a variety of rapidly evolving national and local health-care policy and subsequent legislation changes in relation to NMP. Additionally, there was a requirement to cascade this knowledge to local health-care organisations such as trusts in order to promote service and role redesign to maximise the potential for NMP. The overall strategic aim was to improve access to medicines for patients in a safe and effective manner and ensure that the national targets for training NMP were met.

At the outset of my appointment in the NMP facilitator role the Surrey and Sussex SHA encompassed 28 acute, primary and mental health-care trusts. This did fluctuate during my tenure with some merging of trusts and boundary changes.

From a quantitative perspective, the project role met its primary objectives by increasing the number of qualified NMPs. From a qualitative perspective, it was possible to develop effective systems in order to support the prescribing process and support the CPD needs of all prescribers. Success of the project was further enhanced with partnership, working with all of the trusts that had each appointed a trust NMP lead. I will discuss this in more detail later in this chapter.

The appointment of a NMP facilitator was over a fixed term; originally this was from December 2003 until April 2005. During this period there was rapidly successive legislation changes, until 1 May 2006 when nurses and pharmacists who were qualified and practising as NMPs were enabled to prescribe independently from the whole of the British National Formulary (BNF) (excluding unlicensed medicines and a limited range of controlled drugs) for any medical condition within their sphere of competence (DH 2006). As an outcome of this, the project role was extended until March 2007.

The policy directive to extend prescribing rights also stipulated that organisations must ensure that arrangements are in place for assessment of practice, clinical supervision, audit and monitoring and provide CPD for prescribers.

In spite of this, I was faced with redundancy when the post of NMP facilitator was withdrawn during the merger of Surrey and Sussex SHA with Kent SHA in 2006; I set up independently as a consultant in NMP development and now run my own bespoke NMP CPD workshops and conferences.

My experience in these roles has led to the conclusion that on the whole, CPD for NMPs is not consistently implemented and that demand from NMPs for CPD is not met. For example, a recent workshop on antibiotic prescribing that I organised was oversubscribed with 100 applicants for 40 designated places. Many applicants have commented that there are very little CPD study events available to access. This is a concern because there is a potential that this lack of CPD may lead to ineffective prescribing practice.

SHA Regional NMP facilitators (some SHAs entitled the role 'prescribing lead') were recruited nationally during 2002/3 after the introduction of *Extended Formulary Prescribing* (DH 2002) for nurses and during the introduction of *Supplementary Prescribing for Pharmacists and Nurses* (DH 2003). These developments were quickly followed by the introduction of supplementary prescribing for allied health professionals (DH 2005c).

SHAs were tasked with improving efficient workforce planning and the modernisation of services in direct response to ensuring that patients got faster access to medicines as outlined above and also the implementation of the European Working Time Directive; cutting doctors' working hours but increasing the demand for their expertise had implications for extending the clinical roles and responsibilities of other health-care professionals. The SHA regional NMP facilitators had a key role within these developments.

The SHA regional NMP facilitators' posts were allocated generous budgets to help them in developing NMP across their regions of responsibility. It was crucial for the NMP facilitator to develop productive relationships with NMP leads who had been appointed by the Trusts within the region and assist them in determining and delivering CPD provision, although the extent to which this help was forthcoming depended upon the capacity of each individual SHA facilitator in terms of time, innovation and ability.

When I took up the regional SHA NMP lead role the project had ring-fenced funding directly from Department of Health for several years, which enabled the use of a variety of resources for CPD.

I used these resources in order to develop a database of all regional health-care professionals within training for NMP and those who had already qualified. This included the name of their employing Trust and the job title in which they were undertaking a prescribing role.

I would recommend this approach to anyone who takes responsibility for NMP at the SHA level because I found that it enabled me to identify the most common areas of prescribing practice, and in partnership with the trust NMP leads, plan CPD topics on the basis of this information.

In order to take a cost-effective approach, the content of CPD training needed to be broad enough to be relevant to the majority of NMPs. It proved challenging to plan and develop content for NMPs within highly specialised areas. For example, there was just one pharmacist within the region with an NMP role in treatment for HIV.

The National Prescribing Centre (NPC) has developed high-quality therapeutic workshops for NMPs on a number of relevant topics. Trainers for the workshops are recruited on the basis of being a relevant health-care professional, for example, a pharmacist, and having sound knowledge of therapeutics and clinical epidemiology. The NPC provides training for the workshop facilitators and also the resource materials for the workshops such as PowerPoint slides and reference worksheets. Potential topics that may be offered include asthma, chronic obstructive pulmonary disease (COPD), gastrointestinal conditions, dementia, depression, bacterial infections, palliative care, aural care and dermatology.

The budget allocated by Surrey and Sussex SHA for CPD for NMPs created a possibility for commissioning these on a bi-monthly basis during 2005–2006. I planned for the topics for these by using the information collated on the database to ensure that participants' CPD needs would be met with appropriate workshop content.

Each event was well attended by the regional nurse, pharmacist and allied health professional NMPs and positively evaluated by those who attended it in relation to the content of the workshops.

During 2004, I developed a service development questionnaire in order to identify the sources that individual NMPs were accessing (Figure 4.1). I implemented the questionnaire regionally from 2004–2005. The questionnaire was forwarded to all independent and supplementary nurse prescribers and a random selection of district nurse and health visitor prescribers. A total of 418 completed forms were returned, providing a response rate of 57%. This enabled me to determine the frequency of prescribing by qualified NMPs. Twenty four percent of respondents indicated that they had not written a prescription over the previous 6 months owing to lack of access to appropriate prescription forms.

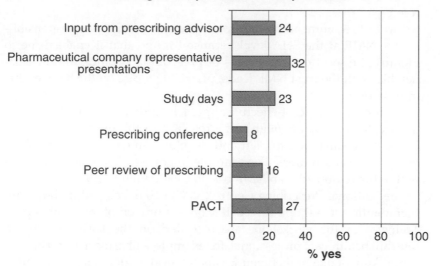

Figure 4.1 Sources of CPD: Outcomes from a service development questionnaire.

The role of Trust NMP leads

As a regional NMP facilitator, I worked very closely with the Trust NMP leads who had been appointed by each of the Trusts within their region. For more discussion about organising CPD for NMP from a Trust perspective, see Chapter 2 and Box 4.2.

Box 4.2 The role of an NHS Trust NMP Lead

> Overall co-ordination of non-medical prescribing agenda within the organisation through the following:
>
> - Monitoring and interpretation of non-medical prescribing activity
> - Provision of specialist advice
> - Assessment of practice, clinical supervision, audit and provision of CPD for non-medical prescribers
> - Integration of clinical governance and risk management procedures with non-medical prescribing
> - Promotion of non-medical prescribing training for relevant staff
> - Support of those undertaking non-medical prescribing training
> - Liaison with education providers.

The NHS Trust NMP leads involved in the project were committed to service redesign and development and to support the implementation of NMP in their locality, reporting to the non-medical local forum.

Organising CPD via a local forum

Having learned a great deal about NMP from national networking, I set up a local forum for the local NHS Trust NMP leads. I chaired and led this forum in order to deliver national progress on NMP and to receive and discuss regional and local issues (Box 4.3). Our local education providers of NMP courses were also invited to the forum in order to forge links and discuss issues such as NMP course application criteria and relevant outcomes for those currently in training.

Box 4.3 Purpose of a local forum for non-medical prescribing

- Networking and sharing ideas for the development of non-medical prescribing
- Identifying a strategy for the development of a non-medical prescribing policy for each NHS trust
- Identifying core principles of the NHS Trust NMP lead role
- Discussing, reviewing and evaluating implemented CPD for non-medical prescribing
- Developing positive marketing strategies for non-medical prescribing
- Reviewing the contribution to service delivery of non-medical prescribing.

During 2005, these meetings were held twice. The Terms of Reference were that the purpose of the group was to identify and develop robust processes for the implementation and development of NMP in each NHS organisation across Surrey and Sussex.

Part of my role was to plan the date and agenda of meetings and to ensure distribution of the minutes. Each set of minutes would contain the relevant action points and who was responsible for achieving identified outcomes and by an agreed date. I understand that these meetings have continued since my departure from the SHA.

At the end of the NMP project, which I had been appointed to lead, I developed a plan to support the Trust NMP leads to take CPD forward in the future.

This led to considerable debate, for example, as to whether or not training organised for CPD should require mandatory participation and whether or not the education providers of NMP (local universities) should also be commissioned to provide CPD.

We identified that the PCT Medicines Management Team had sufficient knowledge to potentially map NPC prescribing competencies with 'intention to treat' by NMPs against the prescribing and cost analysis data (PACT) that they have access to.

It was suggested that the database that had been set up to include the details of regional NMPs could also be used to record, monitor and track attendance at CPD events.

The service development questionnaire, implemented in 2004/2005 and outlined above, revealed that just 2% of respondents indicated that they had received specific performance appraisals about their prescribing practice.

The suggestions that I made in order to overcome this was to link CPD for NMP to *The Knowledge and Skills Framework* (KSF), staff appraisals, personal development plans and Trust NMPs where appropriate. The role of the pharmaceutical industry was also discussed.

Delivering CPD via a local forum

The following section outlines how networking at a national level enabled dissemination of information and support to NHS Trusts in providing CPD for NMPs.

The Trust NMP leads were encouraged to organise a local forum in order to provide qualified NMPs with an opportunity to meet for networking and to contribute towards their CPD needs.

Each Trust decided as to who was most appropriate to be encouraged to attend these events and how they were facilitated. Sometimes it was necessary for these forums to be held out of work hours because the pressure of work commitments did not allow time for meetings during working hours. Not all Trusts had access to funding and sought sponsorship from pharmaceutical companies in order to secure expert speakers relevant to prescribing.

Reflection: providing CPD for non-medical prescribers

Setting up networking events for NMPs within my facilitator lead role within the Surrey and Sussex region and organising my own conferences' feedback from participants has indicated that there are real benefits from talking to one another about individual prescribing practice.

I have used this knowledge in order to facilitate networking sessions within the conferences that I organise. I have developed conference booking forms for participants to state the remit of their prescribing practice so that I can place them in small groups with other participants with similar interests. I suggest that they identify an example of good or effective practice in relation to prescribing within their employing trust. Similarly, I also suggest that they identify a challenging issue in relation to prescribing (Box 4.4).

Box 4.4 Good practice and challenging issues

- The use of clinical management plans for legal prescribing of medicines that are classified as unlicensed when more than one formulation
- Processes to support employers to formulate non-medical prescribing policies in order to identify the remit of prescribing roles, for example, mental health trusts who wished to differentiate between independent and supplementary prescribing roles
- Development of a database of web-based resources to support prescribing practice
- Support of community practitioner nurse prescribers in order to utilise prescribing skills and maintain competence within prescribing practice.

I always include evaluation in the CPD events that I organise and it would appear to me that networking with others is a valued aspect of CPD for NMPs. The reasons for this as stated by participants are given in Box 4.5.

Box 4.5 Feedback from participants attending CPD events for non-medical prescribers

- An opportunity to review what other prescribers are putting into practice
- An opportunity to gather feedback from other prescribers in order to disseminate to other colleagues
- Important to have an opportunity to attend facilitated events where everyone has an opportunity to express their views
- Useful to be placed with participants from similar clinical settings
- An opportunity to share good practice especially for policy and protocol development
- Supportive to realise that other prescribers face similar challenges.

Where are we now?

Since the reduction of 28 SHAs to 10 SHAs within the NHS in England in 2006 as an outcome of organisational change, the funding for NMP has changed.

During 2006/2007, many NHS Trusts had massively overspent and SHAs were required to prune their workforces. A distinct role for an NMP lead facilitator was no longer feasible and it is one of many roles that an individual within the SHA may have to encompass within a comprehensive portfolio of responsibilities. This, I believe, has led to inadequate provision of CPD for NMPs.

During my appointment as regional NMP facilitator for Surrey and Sussex SHA, I attended the monthly NMP briefing meetings chaired and led by the Department of Health. All of the national and regional SHA, NMP facilitators had the opportunity to share progress and information on the development of NMP at a national level. The numbers attending this meeting diminished from 28 SHA regional NMP leads to 10 in line with the number of SHAs in 2006/2007, although the meetings do continue. These meetings, along with national NMP conferences, enabled the SHA regional NMP facilitators to network and share work and ideas on the development of NMP.

Similarly, re-organisation at NHS Trust level has cascaded these issues where the NMP lead role is amongst other pressing challenges of the post holder – for example, also holding responsibility as associate director of nursing, Trust pharmaceutical advisor or Trust head of education and development.

I currently know of just one SHA regional NMP facilitator and one Trust NMP lead nationally whose entire job is devoted to NMP. The impact of this lack of leadership has resulted in inadequate NMP CPD provision generally, although there are some exceptions to this.

A potential solution to this could be the appointment of a national NMP lead with a remit to liaise between the Department of Health and the relevant professional bodies who represent NMPs. This has the potential to identify and develop systems in order to assist SHA and Trust NMP leads within their complex and busy roles.

In the absence of such a role, both regional SHA NMP leads and Trust NMP leads are required to allocate time to sourcing and developing all available resources to build an infrastructure for CPD provision.

The further sections within this chapter will make some suggestions about how this could be achieved.

From 2004–2007, the Department of Health requested quarterly monitoring information in relation to the job/profession category of each non-medical prescriber from each region. As the lead NMP facilitator within the Surrey and Sussex region, it was my responsibility to collect and collate this data regionally. The database, which I set-up and outlined above, provided the information for this purpose.

The Department Health no longer requests this information; however, ideally I would recommend this to anyone in a similar role, in order to collect this data as a basis for planning CPD for NMPs at regional or local level.

The regional NMP lead could build an awareness of the potential for organisations who have resources and expertise to provide CPD for NMPs. For example, HEIs that provide and deliver the NMP courses have developed considerable expertise within NMP and could be commissioned at a regional level to provide CPD prescribing programmes.

It is important to evaluate the quality and cost of various educational approaches and promote accessibility by ensuring that NHS NMP Trust leads are made aware of quality provision and how, where and when it is available.

I developed a business case for the provision of CPD for NMPs within Surrey and Sussex by outlining a range of options and including the benefits, risks, costs, timescales and evaluation of each approach.

The options identified included the allocation of funding, the commissioning of CPD by a variety of providers, the allocation of funding to provide each Trust with their own CPD trainer and the option to do nothing.

The option of implementing mandatory CPD was discussed, but it was decided that it would be too complex to oversee and maintain. For example, what action could be taken if NMPs did not access their mandatory CPD, would they then be excluded from actively prescribing, and what pathway would enable them to prescribe in the future, and who would oversee this?

This is an important debate for regional NMP leads to engage in, especially within the context of recent recommendations for CPD that professional bodies have made (NMC 2008; RPSGB 2007).

An appraisal should always be made in order to determine the quality of education. The level of knowledge of the trainer could be established by checking educational qualifications and whether or not they access to up to date and evidence-based information. The job title of the trainer will not necessarily ensure quality and that includes senior medical staff.

It is also important to take into account that individuals will have different learning styles and it is important to offer a diversity of educational approaches. The various chapters within this book offer a variety of suggestions.

Some NHS Trusts may have their own in-house training for NMPs, some will use external speakers, some will have a local HEI that provides CPD and some will have no provision at all.

Commissioning CPD for non-medical prescribers

With the separation of commissioner and provider roles within PCTs and increased bureaucracy in agreeing contracts, there may be confusion regarding commissioning and providing CPD, which may result in delayed or no delivery.

It is a dichotomy to invest in training individuals within the NHS to qualify as NMPs and then not fund CPD education to support and sustain this.

I would recommend that anyone who has a Trust lead role for NMP submits a business case to the regional NMP lead in order to secure annual funding for CPD. By undertaking a local training analysis of the CPD needs of NMP, they would be well placed to commission and evaluate appropriate education and ensure value for money.

The NMC standards for CPD for NMPs (2008) state that each NMP should have a personal development plan in place, which includes an analysis of individual training and education needs. This information could also be used to undertake a scoping and mapping exercise to plan training and education at a local and regional level (Box 4.6). This could then be developed to include timescales for the implementation of training and a projection of likely costs.

Box 4.6 Suggested project plan for meeting CPD training needs for non-medical prescribers at a regional level

---

- Using information from individual personal development plans (PDPs), identify current professional roles of local non-medical prescribers.
- Identify and cost potential local sources, which can meet training needs of non-medical prescribers.
- Identify a specific time period for implementation of training.
- Develop a plan for evaluation of the project.

The advantages of this approach is that it takes into account the current remit of roles of NMPs and makes it possible to consider how these roles might develop in the future.

The outcome should enable the regional NMP lead to plan and resource future (CPD) training provisions to equip a NMP workforce fit for practice within the NHS.

Within the Surrey and Sussex region, the findings of a commissioned training needs analysis of CPD for NMPs (Green 2006) demonstrated that short courses (1-day or 2-day) that were specific to the NMPs role were generally considered to be the most popular and useful.

When planning training events they do need to be advertised well in advance (at least 6 weeks' notice) in order that potential participants are able to arrange workload and other commitments around a programme of their choice. In addition, clarity of the learning outcomes on the advertising literature by the education provider is always helpful for the potential to enable them to make their choices.

Conclusion

In this chapter, I have reflected on my personal experience in order to convey my perspective that the current provision of CPD for NMP needs investment in time and money in order to develop.

In the meantime, it is the responsibility of those who lead on the development of NMP at the regional and organisational level to ensure that their NMPs have systems in place to help them access training to help them maintain and improve their standard of prescribing practice. This chapter has provided a few examples of what has worked well and lessons learned based on my own personal experience.

Key learning points

- The *New Labour* health-care policy agenda identified new roles for professionals working within the NHS, which included non-medical prescribing.
- Many regional health-care organisations were provided with ring-fenced budgets in order to support the development of non-medical prescribing, which included the appointment of non-medical prescribing lead roles at the regional level. This role was identified in order to develop training programmes and CPD for non-medical prescribing.
- Lead roles for non-medical prescribing were also identified at the NHS trust level.
- Many primary objectives were achieved in that numbers of qualified non-medical prescribers increased.
- The objectives for CPD for non-medical prescribers were less clearly identified.
- Since the reduction in numbers of regional health-care organisations within the United Kingdom, regional non-medical prescribing roles have diminished.
- This has resulted in less infrastructure for CPD for non-medical prescribers.
- In regions where CPD for non-medical prescribing has been supported and developed a core success factor is a regional and local training needs analysis.
- New directives for CPD for non-medical prescribers (RPSGB 2008; NMC 2008) have outlined a framework of requirements.
- In spite of these, CPD for non-medical prescribers is not consistently implemented and demand for CPD for non-medical prescribing is not met.
- A regional training needs analysis of CPD for non-medical prescribing can form the basis of a business plan in order to commission CPD.

Key resources in Section Three

- Useful websites
- Practical advice for organisation of CPD for non-medical prescribers.
- Practical advice for facilitation of CPD for non-medical prescribers.

References

Department of Health (1999) *NSF for Mental Health: Modern Standards and Service Models*. London, Department of Health.

Department of Health (2000) *The NHS Plan: A Plan for Investment, a Plan for Reform*. London, Department of Health.

Department of Health (2002) *Extending Independent Nurse Prescribing in the NHS in England. A Guide for Implementation*. London, Department of Health.

Department of Health (2003) *Supplementary Prescribing by Nurses and Pharmacists within the NHS in England. A Guide for Implementation*. London, Department of Health.

Department of Health (2004) *The NHS Improvement Plan, Putting People at the Heart of Public Services*. London, Department of Health.

Department of Health (2005a) *Supporting People with Long Term Conditions. An NHS and Social Care Model to Support Local Innovation and Integration*. London, Department of Health.

Department of Health (2005b) *Creating a Patient-Led NHS: Delivering the NHS Improvement Plan*. London, Department of Health.

Department of Health (2005c) *Supplementary Prescribing by Nurses, Physiotherapists, Chiropodists, Podiatrists and Radiographers within the NHS in England: A Guide for Implementation*. London, Department of Health.

Department of Health (2006) *Extending Independent Nurse Prescribing in England: A Guide for Implementation*. London, Department of Health.

Green, A. (2006) *Provision of Continuing Professional Development for Nurses & Pharmacists within the Surrey and Sussex Strategic Health Authority for Non-medical Prescribers – a Training Needs Analysis*. (Unpublished Project Report).

Nursing and Midwifery Council (2008) *Guidance for Continuing Professional Development for Nurse and Midwife Prescribers*. London, NMC.

Royal Pharmaceutical Society of Great Britain (2007) *Clinical Governance Framework for Pharmacist Prescribers and Organisations Commissioning or Participating in Pharmacist Prescribing*. London, RPGSB.

Section Two

Specific Approaches to CPD for Non-Medical Prescribers

5 Using E-learning for CPD within Non-Medical Prescribing

Marion Waite

Introduction

This chapter is a practical guide to planning continuing professional development (CPD) for non-medical prescribers, supported by the use of learning technologies. It has been written on the basis of experience in the use of learning technologies to support non-medical prescribing training and an evaluation project, which was undertaken in order to establish some best practice guidance for National Health Service (NHS) organisations when developing e-learning for CPD for health-care professionals (Waite & Bingham 2008).

The chapter outlines how to go about embedding learning technologies within the organisation and also reviews current online resources that are accessible for non-medical prescribers in order to support CPD. This is potentially of interest to the individual non-medical prescriber, who may be organising their own CPD, or managers at either trust or regional level, who have a role to support non-medical prescribers. Listed in Box 5.1 are terms associated with learning technologies.

Box 5.1 Glossary of terms associated with learning technologies

Blended learning – a combination of traditional teaching approaches and e-learning.

Blog – a shortening of the word web log, which is a website where entries are commonly displayed in reverse chronological order. 'Blog' can also be used as a verb, meaning to maintain or add content to more personal online diaries.

DfES – Department for Education and Skills http://www.dfes.gov.uk/.

Digital repositories – hold a wide range of materials for a variety of purposes and users in order to support research and learning. They can help to manage institutions' intellectual assets.

E-learning – the JISC definition of e-learning is 'learning facilitated and supported through the use of information and communications technology'. This definition has been broadly adopted throughout the education research community.

E-portfolio – an electronically based portfolio, which is a file storage and information management system modelled on the working method used for paper portfolios, but which takes advantage of the capabilities of ICT, notably allowing learners to store digital artefacts and streamlining the process of review and moderation for learners and educators.

ICT – Information Communications Technology.

JISC – Joint Information Systems Committee. An independent advisory body that works with further and higher education by providing strategic guidance, advice and opportunities to use ICT to support learning and teaching. http://www.jisc.ac.uk/.

KSF – Knowledge and Skills Framework.

MLE – Managed Learning Environment. A range of different software, systems and processes that interrelate, share data and contribute to the management of the learner experience within an organisation.

MP3 files – an audio or video file that is downloadable to a mobile device or computer.

Mobile-learning – a variant of e-learning where the learning is undertaken using a mobile ICT device (e.g. a PDA, mobile phone, hand-held computer, etc.).

PDA – Personal digital assistant.

PDP – Personal development plan.

Podcast – a collection of digital media files that is distributed over the Internet, often using syndication feeds, for playback on portable media players and personal computers. The term podcast, like 'broadcast', can refer either to the series of content itself or to the method by which it is syndicated.

Skype – software program that allows users to make telephone calls over the Internet to other Skype users free of charge and to landlines and cell phones for a fee. Additional features include instant messaging, file transfer, short message service, video conferencing and the ability to circumvent firewalls.

VLE – Virtual Learning Environment, which consists of a set of learning and teaching tools based within a local network that consists of content, resources and learning activities. Standard functions include curriculum mapping, learner tracking, communication tools, tutor and learner support, assessment and learning delivery tools.

> **Wiki –** software that allows users to easily create, edit, and link pages. Wikis are often used to create collaborative websites and to power community websites. These wiki websites are often also referred to as *wikis*; for example, Wikipedia is one of the best-known wikis. The word wiki is derived from the Haiiwan word for fast.

Background

The Joint Information Systems Committee (JISC; http://www.jisc.ac.uk) is a UK government funded body, which has been set up in order to provide leadership within education and research and the use of information communication technologies. The JISC defines *e-learning* as 'learning facilitated and supported through the use of information and communications technology'. This definition has been generally adopted throughout the education research community. This is clearly a broad definition and suggests that e-learning is a concept that can involve a wide range of communication and information technologies.

Blended learning, which can use e-learning as a component, has emerged globally as an important mechanism for delivering CPD education in a range of work place and academic settings. Bonk & Graham (2006) have described blended learning as 'the most prominent delivery mechanism in higher education, business, government and military settings'. This can be attributed to the developments in technology and the potential for flexible learning opportunities. It is widely acknowledged that blended learning is poorly defined and broadly interpreted (Bonk & Graham 2006; Sharpe *et al.* 2006). Collis *et al.* (2005) liken blended learning to the distinction between formal and informal learning: the former is planned and structured, whereas the latter is more likely to happen in the workplace, based on experience and in conjunction with peers. The ideal blend makes the most of both of these. For example, non-medical prescribers could plan a formal teaching session where they taught the theoretical use of the British National Formulary (BNF) to a student prescriber with some practical exercises and informally demonstrated this to the student in practice whilst making a prescribing decision. The learner would have experienced a learning blend.

In practical terms, however, the most common notion of blended learning is traditional face-to-face teaching, which is supported by a range of learning technologies such as online resources and learning modules, and also with the integration of newer technologies.

Ryan *et al.* (2000) have highlighted the trends that global competition has created in industrialised countries for lifelong learning and more flexible career options. This has, in turn, encouraged the development of strategies for blended learning and e-learning in order to respond to these trends.

Government policy documents such as *Making a Difference* (DH 1999) and *The NHS Plan* (DH 2000) outlined the commitment to CPD within the NHS and the need to support existing staff in order to meet clinical governance requirements and develop their roles. The *Knowledge and Skills Framework* (KSF) (DH 2003) describes the skills that NHS staff need in order to carry out their roles competently. Although the KSF does not relate directly to non-medical prescribing, the *NMC Standards of Proficiency for Non-Medical Prescribers* (NMC 2006) have set standards for practice and education and a recent addition to this is the *Guiding Principles for CPD for nurse and Midwife Prescribers* (NMC 2008).

A multitude of trends within educational, information and communication technologies have implications for the future of CPD education within the NHS. Bury *et al.* (2006) have commented on an information-rich and technological age, which is influencing health information professionals within the NHS.

A survey carried out by the National Prescribing Centre (NPC) (NPC 2007) found that 53% of non-medical prescribers registered with their network and that 75% of their managers felt that e-learning had a place within their CPD.

Supporting Best Practice in E-learning across the NHS (DH 2005) sets out a national strategy to promote e-learning as a tool to improve accessibility to education for all health-care staff. It recognises that there is a need to build capacity and capability for e-learning within the NHS and recommends that this can be encouraged by highlighting examples of good practice. Success is dependent on robust mechanisms for delivery, quality content and resources, the preparedness of learners and the ability and flexibility of managers and practice educators to support learners. This can be underpinned with local strategic leadership and effective change management.

Examples of e-learning initiatives that have been implemented at a national level within the NHS include the Core Learning Unit Programmes, which provide standardised and quality-assured e-modules for mandatory training and E-learning for Healthcare (e-LFH), which aims to deliver e-learning modules for health-care professionals and a soon-to-be-launched managed learning environment (MLE) for staff who work for NHS professionals to encompass statutory and mandatory modules.

The e-LFH project is based on a model that has worked well for radiographers and is a good example of collaborative working with a professional body to deliver CPD education. All of the above initiatives are very recent and it is not clear how uptake and success will be evaluated in the long term. Furthermore, they rely purely on online delivery, yet blended learning is the preferred option for many CPD learners. This has implications for NHS organisations trying to encourage access and uptake. Moreover, the reality of life as an NHS professional means not having a permanent practice base and this may minimise access to technology for online modules.

The E-KSF (http://www.e-ksfnow.org/) is an online tool to help NHS organisations and health-care professionals to implement the KSF and relate it to individual personal development plan (PDP) processes. This shows great potential for future developments, especially the integration of e-portfolios. The Electronic Staff Record (ESR) (http://www.esrsolution.co.uk) is a human resource tool, which will be linked to the NHS payroll system, and a module of this will detail and record the ongoing training and education of individuals. In addition, a national learning management system (NLMS) will be an optional link to the ESR and will provide NHS staff with access to e-learning resources and programmes offered at a national level. The NLMS is due to be rolled out from September 2008.

NHS Connecting for Health (http://www.connectingforhealth.nhs.uk) supports implementation of the National Programme for IT and a crucial strand of this includes education, training and development for NHS staff. These developments will no doubt encourage the building of e-learning skills for health-care professionals such as non-medical prescribers, but this will take time to implement and the NHS is currently in a transitory phase in relation to these.

Modernising Health Care Training (DH 2006) sets out a road map for e-learning within the NHS and has led to the formation of the UK Alliance for E-learning Partners, which is a collaboration of key stakeholders from the NHS and professional bodies who represent a range of health-care professionals who work in the NHS. It recognises the need to develop learning infrastructures and systems so that more NHS staff can access e-learning and maximise learning in the workplace. An NHS e-learning objects repository is currently being implemented with the aim of providing NHS organisations with access to a digital repository of downloadable e-learning resources.

How can learning technologies be used in practice?

So, how can the busy NHS manager or trust learning-lead plan blended learning within their organisation to meet the CPD needs of non-medical prescribers?

Motivation to participate is best when health-care professionals can relate the planned learning to what they want to learn. The use of personal development plans and competency frameworks such as the NPC *Competency Framework* can help to identify individual learning needs. In reality, a professional who has successfully completed the non-medical prescribing course is likely to have a good idea about how he or she would like to further advance their prescribing practice. This should help to guide the instructor in the planning and identification of appropriate resources and designing learning activities that meet these needs.

Competency-based assessment is relevant for CPD for all health-care professionals and e-learning is considered to offer potential for a more standardised approach. Other potential advantages are considered to be cost-effectiveness and provision of timely and equitable access to training materials. Clearly, there is a challenge of balancing service needs with educational needs and a lack of clearly defined competencies for e-learning.

Candy (2008) has outlined six principles in relation to the needs for successful implementation of *Connecting for Health* but has made the point that it is important to also consider what can be learned from e-learning developments outside of the NHS. He particularly highlights the benefits of NHS collaboration with other organisations such as HEIs and FE colleges in order to work in partnership to create learning strategies and resources and avoid duplication and unwanted variation.

There is an increasing number of good examples of peer-reviewed online resources ranging from complete online modules to digital repositories that store learning objects, which can be downloaded and adapted to the needs of the user.

If you are planning to implement blended learning within your organisation, it is more likely to be successful if you engage support from senior management and other technical staff who have skills in facilitating the use of learning technologies and accessing information, especially NHS librarians. Although blended learning is deemed to be flexible, examples where it has worked well suggest that participants and instructors need to have protected time in order to carry the activities out and also need to have confidence and accessibility to the technologies that plan to be used.

Collaboration with other organisations such as other trusts and local higher education institutions with relevant experience maximises resources and the use of expertise.

Learning activities, which have relevance to professional practice, especially those that raise ethical and practice-based issues are more likely to be effective. Lacey-Bryant & Ringrose (2005) have estimated that e-learning contributes to 70% of CPD for general practitioners (GPs) and cite the example of http://www.doctors.net as a good example of a resource that has been developed in conjunction with the Royal

Colleges and contains clinical topic modules, which once completed, can be used to contribute to a PDP.

Using a virtual learning environment (VLE)

A virtual learning environment (VLE) is a platform that enables access to an electronic learning environment, which requires an Internet connection. A VLE is web-based and is a good example within the NHS is the soon-to-be launched MLE. A VLE is housed within a local network and consists of content, resources and learning activities. Standard functions include curriculum mapping, learner tracking, communication tools, tutor and learner support, assessment and learning delivery tools. A VLE enables technology-based learning to be located within one space and for communication between participants and facilitators. For the manager who may have a responsibility to support or develop e-learning, there are a range of VLES that can be downloaded for free from the Internet; a good example is Moodle: (http://moodle.org), which can be used to create an online learning site.

The advantage of using a VLE is that access to CPD can potentially be provided to wide groups of learners over several geographical locations. A VLE can also be used for collaboration and communication, which provides opportunities for shared and collective learning and support. It is also possible to develop web-based resources that are well presented and do not necessitate the need to have in-depth skills or knowledge of web design.

Software such as WImba Create http://www.wimba.com/products/wimba_create/ enables the facilitator or educator to create learning modules that can be uploaded to a VLE from word documents.

Planning a blended learning activity

The Joint Information Systems Committee (JISC) (http://www.jisc.ac.uk) principally supports the work of further and higher education. They also provide a good selection of resources that can be used and adapted to support the uses of technology within education in any setting.

An example is the *Effective Practice Planner*. When designing blended learning the educator is recommended to plan learning activities, explicitly outlining what the learner is expected to do or complete in order to achieve the intended learning outcomes (Table 5.1). Tools such as the Effective Practice Planner can be helpful in this respect.

Table 5.1   Designing an e-learning activity

Issues to consider	Designing a learning activity to incorporate ILT or e-learning
1. Learners (their needs, motives for learning, prior experience of learning, social and interpersonal skills, preferred learning styles and ICT competence)	Qualified non-medical prescribers who specialise in diabetes care who wish to reach consensus about making rational prescribing decisions about new therapies, which have been licensed for the treatment of type 2 diabetes
2. Intended learning outcome (acquisition of knowledge, academic and social skills, increased motivation and ability to progress)	The activity is designed to advance the learners' knowledge about new pharmacological therapies for the treatment of type 2 diabetes, for example, incretin mimetics It is also intended that they will utilise online technologies in order to find relevant information and disseminate their learning to other colleagues It is also hoped that it will further their confidence in searching for evidence and appraisal of this evidence and application to ongoing prescribing practice
3. Learning environment (face to face or virtual) – available resources, tools, facilities and services and their match with the learners' needs	**Where does the activity take place?** In a trust seminar room **What resources are available?** • Word documents or e-books that contain a therapy appraisal framework • Online access to a range of searchable academic and health-care databases with access to published research • A selection of appropriate case histories for discussion and application of new knowledge **What technologies are available?** Data projector and laptop, computer workstations with Internet access for the participants **What features of established practice will be important?** Practitioners' (participants') expert knowledge of topic and content, practice and interpersonal skills. Opportunities are provided for discussion and peer review of new knowledge with face-to-face feedback where required **What support will you require?** Require assistance from trust librarians to provide or refresh knowledge about searching online databases. Assistance from the technical support team to ensure that the equipment is available in the classroom and is functioning

Table 5.1 (*Continued*)

Issues to consider	Designing a learning activity to incorporate ILT or e-learning
4. The learning activity (the means by which the practitioner brings about learning and seeks to influence the development of the learners)	**Describe the learning activity** Activities combining both established and e-learning practice promote the development of critical appraisal skills and allow practitioners to check their own understanding in a safe environment in order to support their decision-making within practice Learners will then be encouraged to compile a PowerPoint presentation that summarises their knowledge and clinical application of therapies for the treatment of type 2 diabetes, which can be shared with other practice-based colleagues The PowerPoint could either be uploaded online to the trust intranet or posted on a WIKI in order to summarise the learning outcomes of the session
5. The approach taken (related to learners' needs, preferred learning styles, the nature of the learning environment and the intended outcomes)	**Learning styles** Searching for and appraising evidence will suit reflective learners. The learners are also actively engaged through their use of the data projector and laptop, encouraging the kinaesthetic learners. Facilitation of discussion can further assist learners with an auditory preference **Inclusion** All practitioners will be actively engaged in the classroom activities. The construction of the PowerPoint is used to get practitioners more actively involved in learning, with facilitators encouraging learners to contribute **Assessment** Formative assessment activities in the form of quizzes and case histories leading to enable learners to check and share their own learning **ILT or e-learning in practice** In a lesson, learners must search and find relevant information that relates to empirical evidence about the use of therapies in the treatment of type 2 diabetes. The facilitator should support the group to decide when a sufficient amount of resources have been located. The searches are saved in order to link with the next activity In the next activity, the facilitator encourages the learners to download the therapy appraisal framework. The group is split into sub-groups in order to review one of the retrieved information sources in relation to the framework The groups share their appraisals and reach a consensus about the role of therapies for the treatment of type 2 diabetes

(*continued overleaf*)

Table 5.1 *(Continued)*

Issues to consider	Designing a learning activity to incorporate ILT or e-learning
	The group use their findings in order to develop a web-based module that summarises the learning outcomes of the session and implications for future prescribing practice
6. How would you evaluate the effectiveness of this learning activity?	**Does this activity engage learners in the learning process?** Yes, all learners have the opportunity to participate through the use of the appraisal framework and group discussion, and the facilitator encourages each member to contribute to the development of a learning resource
	Does this activity encourage independent learning skills? Not directly during the learning activities but it will enhance the development of critical appraisal skills, which will support their independent prescribing decisions
	Does this activity develop learners' skills and knowledge? Yes, learners gain essential skills and improve their knowledge through active participation in the learning activities. The focused class activity ensures full participation in each lesson and allows the tutor to track learner responses and monitor individual progress
	Does this activity motivate further learning? ILT or e-learning in practice There is potential to develop confidence for non-medical prescribers to develop transferable skills such as searching and appraising for evidence and confidence with learning technologies that will help motivate them to learn with these methods in the future

When things do not go well

The factor that contributes to the lack of effectiveness within blended learning is a perception of the lack of participation of some learners by others who have contributed. This is particularly true when using online discussions. The facilitator has an important role in preparing learners so that they may feel confident and competent in order to participate. Salmon (2004) provides a good model, which is a useful resource when planning education involving learning technologies.

There is also evidence to suggest (Waite & Bingham 2008) that orientation to learning technologies can be resource intensive for both the facilitator and the learner, so it is important that protected time is allocated for the development of this.

It is also important to ensure that learning objects and resources are up to date and include references to valid professional guidelines and expertise where relevant.

Web 2.0 technologies

Web 2.0 technologies is the term that is used (Wikipedia 2009) to describe the increasing trend of the use of the World Wide Web, especially for social networking and information sharing.

It is important to consider the potential use of these when implementing blended learning into an organisation. It is also important to consider the use of other formats where there might be problems with access to virtual learning environments such as digital video discs.

A podcast is a collection of digital media files that is distributed over the Internet, often using syndication feeds, for playback on portable media players and personal computers. The term podcast, like 'broadcast', can refer either to the series of content itself or to the method by which it is syndicated. Some universities are beginning to use podcasts for learner feedback and dissemination of lecture content.

An MP3 file is an audio or video file, which is downloadable to a mobile device, this makes for very accessible learning. All of these methods are equally transferable to an NHS setting and are useful considerations for providing CPD to non-medical prescribers.

Boulous *et al.* (2006) suggest that, given the popularity of hand-held devices, mobile-learning has great potential for genuine anywhere, anytime-learning. Devices are easy to use, relatively cheap and easy to implement. Podcasts can be ideal for the busy health-care professional and high-resolution sound definition makes this an ideal format for clinical practice teaching, which relates to a non-medical prescribing role, for example, heart and respiratory sounds.

For the NHS organisation that has an established infrastructure for online learning, it is useful to consider the integration of Web 2.0 technologies.

Mason (2005) suggests that the use of blogs can promote critical thinking and inspire lifelong learning. Blog is a shortening of the word web log, which is a website where entries are commonly displayed in reverse chronological order. 'Blog' can also be used as a verb, meaning to maintain or add content to more personal online diaries. This could be a useful format for a community of non-medical prescribers within an organisation in order to keep up to date with a range of clinical and professional topics. For example, a recent group of learners on one of our prescribing courses set up a blog in order to share their developing knowledge of pharmacology as applied to prescribing practice (Box 5.2).

Box 5.2 How to set up a blog

> - Go to https://www.blogger.com/start.
> - Set up an account.
> - You can chose the design and layout of your blog.
> - You can decide to either keep your blog private by inviting members only or you can leave it open, which means that it may be 'googled' and found by anyone. You also have options about sharing authorship of your blog.

Wiki is a software that allows users to easily create, edit and link pages together. Wikis are often used to create collaborative websites and to power community websites. These Wiki websites are often also referred to as *Wikis*; for example, Wikipedia is one of the best-known Wikis. The word Wiki is derived from the Haiiwan word for fast. Boulous *et al.* (2006) make the point that all technologies require moderation and monitoring, which has implications for the manager or education lead. For example, anyone with access to a Wiki can edit the content, which can lead to issues about reliability. However, the advantage of Wikis is that they are easily updated and are thus potentially very helpful for educational use within fast-changing areas of clinical practice such as non-medical prescribing.

Electronic portfolios

The Nursing and Midwifery Council (NMC) suggests (NMC 2008) that nurse and midwife prescribers record evidence of their CPD within a portfolio. Non-medical prescribers will have been assessed via a portfolio within their initial prescribing training.

Electronic or e-portfolios are an electronically based portfolio, which is a file store and information management system that is modelled on the working method used for paper portfolios, but which takes advantage of the capabilities of ICT, notably allowing learners to store digital artifacts and streamlining the process of review and moderation for learners and educators (JISC 2008).

Whitsed (2005) makes the point that there is no agreed definition of an e-portfolio but concurs with others (Johnson & Davies 2005) that they are associated with lifelong learning and a new and innovative way to collect, manipulate and present material.

The Department for Education and Skills (DFES 2005) proposes a personal online learning space for every learner, which will contribute to an electronic portfolio, building a record of achievement for lifelong learning. This will start during school education.

Learners have found (Mason *et al.* 2004) that the use of an e-portfolio helps them reflect on their skills and competencies and enables them to present them in a format that is readily available to university admissions staff and employers. Learners have also found that they facilitate personal development planning, promote self-direction (Mason *et al.* 2004), present work for academic and work-based assessment and link to Curriculum Vitae.

E-portfolios have potential as key tools to support CPD for non-medical prescribers. This could meet the NMC requirements for the maintenance of a portfolio and enable the prescriber to share their achievements with their employers.

E-portfolios are an important component for the medical foundation programme within the United Kingdom, so are already in use within the NHS. At the organisational level, it is important to consider how these could be developed for wider use. More information about e-portfolios can be found at http://www.jiscinfonet.ac.uk/infokits/e-portfolios.

Review of National Prescribing Centre online resources for non-medical prescribers

Recent guidance (NMC 2008) about CPD and non-medical prescribing leaves no doubt that the individual is responsible for ensuring that their prescribing skills remain up-to-date. So how can the busy non-medical prescriber make the most of online resources, which have been developed in order to support this?

The NPC was established in 1996 by the Department of Health in order to provide information to prescribers about medicines management. The NPC (http://www.npc.co.uk/index.htm) is a very important online resource for non-medical prescribers and contains sections on medicines management, evidence-based therapeutics, policy and supporting prescribers.

A range of publications are available from the website, which includes MeReC Bulletins, which are regularly published in order to bring together all of the available evidence on a range of therapeutic interventions.

NPCI is an interactive online learning resource within the NPC website for prescribers and their managers. A range of Web 2.0 technologies such as blogs and podcasts are effectively utilised in order to deliver relevant learning content. This is a superb resource for CPD and a good introduction to using Web 2.0 for those who are unsure about the possibilities.

The supporting prescribers section contains a sub-section for non-medical prescribers, which includes useful web links for prescribers, competency frameworks, a bi-monthly newsletter Connecting *Prescribers* and an opportunity to join a national network for prescribers.

Other online resources

Although not directly related to prescribing, the following resources are useful to support CPD for non-medical prescribers (also see the resources section of this book).

Onmedica is an online resource that is aimed at doctors, nurses, pharmacists, practice managers and health-care students. Onmedica consists of learning modules, journal articles, blogs and is updated on a daily basis. It is free for all health-care staff who are professionally registered. It also contains an individual personal learning plan, which enables the practitioners to record their learning achievements within the site: http://www.onmedica.com/.

For the BMJ Learning online CPD modules for doctors, nurses, practice managers, GP registrars and other health-care professionals, a subscription is required. This is available either on an individual or institution basis. The latter could be provided by a health-care organisation such as a trust, which will enable them to fulfil their obligation by providing access to CPD resources: http://learning.bmj.com/learning/main.html.

GP Notebook is an online encyclopedia of medicine that provides a trusted immediate reference resource for clinicians in the United Kingdom such as non-medical prescribers: http://www.gpnotebook.co.uk/homepage.cfm.

Building and sharing your own database of online prescribing resources

Social software provides great potential for building a personal database of resources and interacting and sharing these with an online community with similar interests.

In particular, social bookmarking is a form of free social software that uses a 'tagging' system to discover or share web-based bookmarks (OCSLD 2008).

An example is Delicious (http://delicious.com/). We encourage participants within our prescribing courses to create a personal 'delicious' account. This enables them to store all of their relevant prescribing bookmarks in one place and share them amongst the group, if they wish. This is done creating a tag that is agreed by the course cohort, for example, 'nmp JAN08'. This creates endless possibilities for sharing relevant website, journal articles and outputs from database searches, which relate to prescribing. Other free social bookmarking sites include Facebook, Stumbleupon and DIGG IT!

Conclusion

The continued development of learning technologies has a clear role to play within CPD for non-medical prescribers. This has implications for both the individual non-medical prescriber and their employing organisation.

The busy manager is advised to consider how they can embed learning technologies within the organisation and have an awareness of what the possibilities are for their use. It is also important to create access to learning technologies and facilitate and support staff, so that they can make the most of the potential possibilities.

The individual non-medical prescriber is professionally responsible for keeping their prescribing practice up to date and this includes identifying valid and reliable resources in order to support this. Some online resources are already available and familiarisation with these is highly recommended for the non-medical prescriber. In addition, the use of social bookmarking sites can enable the non-medical prescriber to build and share their own repository of technology-enhanced resources in order to support their CPD.

Key learning points

- E-learning is a concept that can involve a wide range of learning technologies.
- Blended learning has emerged as a global trend within CPD and consists of a combination of face-to-face teaching supported by a range of learning technologies.
- A range of initiatives within the NHS have implications for e-learning and this has implications for non-medical prescribers and their managers.
- The use of Web 2.0 technologies and e-portfolios are important for developing, building and sharing resources, which have relevance to non-medical prescribing.
- Valid and reliable online resources, which relate to non-medical pre-scribing directly and indirectly, are freely available and accessible.

Key resources in Section Three

- Useful websites, with critique
- JISC Effective E-learning Planner.

References

Bonk, C. J. and Graham, C. R. (Eds) (2006) *The Handbook of Blended Learning: Global Perspectives, Local Designs*. San Francisco, Pfeiffer.

Boulous, M., Maramba, I. and Wheeler, S. (2006) Wikis, blogs & pod casts: a new generation of web-based tools for virtual collaborative clinical practice and education. *BMC Medical Education* 6: 41.

Bury, R., Martin, L. and Roberts, S. (2006) Achieving change through mutual development: supported online-learning and the evolving roles of health and information professionals. *Health Information and Libraries Journal* 23 (Suppl.1): 22–31.

Candy, P. (2008) 2nd NESC e-learning communication and consultation event; Conference Proceedings, Newbury, March 31st 2008.

Collis, B., Bianco, M., Margrayan, A. and Waring, B. (2005) Putting blended learning to work: a case study from a multinational oil company. *Education, Information and Information* 5(3): 135–142.

DFES (2005) *The e-Strategy Harnessing Technology: Transforming Learning and Children's Services*. London, Department for Education and Skills, Children, Schools and Families.

DH (1999) *Making a Difference: Strengthening the Nursing, Midwifery and Health Visiting Contribution to Healthcare*. London, Department of Health.

DH (2000) *The NHS Plan*. London, Department of Health.

DH (2003) *The NHS Knowledge and Skills Framework (NHS KSF)*. London, Department of Health.

DH (2005) *Supporting Best Practice in E-learning across The NHS*. London, Department of Health.

DH (2006) *Modernising Healthcare Training: E-learning in Healthcare Services*. London, The Department of Health.

JISC (2008) http://www.jisc.ac.uk/whatwedo/themes/elearning/eportfolios.aspx [Accessed 17 April 2009].

Johnson, M. and Davies, S. (2005) *How Can You Pilot Lifelong Learning? The Experiences of the JISC Distributed E-learning Regional Pilot Projects*. Bolton, University of Bolton, JISC. http://www.jisc.ac.uk/media/documents/programmes/capital/boltonbidr.pdf.

Lacey-Bryant, S. and Ringrose, T. (2005) Evaluating the Doctors.net UK model of electronic continuing medical education. *Work Based Learning in Primary Care* 3: 129–142.

Mason, R. (2005) Guest editorial – blended learning. *Education, Communications and Information* 5(3): 356–372.

Mason, R., Peglar, C. and Weller, M. (2004) E-portfolios: an assessment tool for online courses. *British Journal of Educational Technology* 35(6): 42–46.

Nursing and Midwifery Council (2006) *Standards of Proficiency for Nurse and Midwife Prescribers*. London, NMC.

Nursing and Midwifery Council (2008) *Guidance for Continuing Professional Development for Nurse and Midwife Prescribers*. London, NMC.

NPC (2007) *Results of Surveying Non Medical Prescribers*. Liverpool, The National Prescribing Centre.

OCSLD (2008) *Oxford Centre for Staff Learning and Development*. Oxford, Oxford Brookes University.

Ryan, S., Scott, B., Freeman, H. and Patel, D. (2000) *The Virtual University – The Internet and Resource-Based Learning*. London, Kogan Page.

Salmon, G. (2004) *e-Moderating. The Key to Teaching and Learning Online*, 2nd edition. Abingdon, Routledge.

Sharpe, R., Benfield, G., Roberts, G. and Francis, R. (2006) *The Undergraduate Experience of Blended E-learning: A Review of UK Literature and Practice*. Oxford, Higher Education Academy.

Waite, M. and Bingham, H. (2008) *Best Practice Guidance for Blended Learning Approaches to CPD for Education for NHS Staff*. Newbury, NHS Education South Central.

Whitsed (2005) E-portfolios an introduction. *Learning and Teaching*.

Wikipedia http://en.wikipedia.org/wiki/Web_2.0 [Accessed 20 February 2009].

Useful websites

https://www.blogger.com/start

http://www.connectingforhealth.nhs.uk

http://delicious.com/

http://www.doctors.net

http://www.dfes.gov.uk/

http://e-ksfnow.org/

http://www.esrsolution.co.uk

http://www.gpnotebook.co.uk/homepage.cfm

http://www.jisc.ac.uk/

http://www.jiscinfonet.ac.uk/infokits/e-portfolios

http://learning.bmj.com/learning/main.html

http://moodle.org/

http://www.npc.co.uk/index.htm

http://www.onmedica.com/

http://www.wimba.com/products/wimba_create/

6 Action Learning and Learning Sets

Jan Keenan

Introduction

The concept of reflection is not new to the health professions, and it has proved a useful learning tool in both formal and informal settings. This chapter sets out some of the theory in relation to learning from reflection and action, through action learning, and applies some of this theory to generate ideas for developing action learning-based approaches to continuing professional development (CPD) for non-medical prescribers.

Action learning

Action learning is a process of reflection and action, aimed at improving the effectiveness of action where learning is an important outcome (Bourner 1996 cited in Koo 1999). To put in simple terms, it is a description of how most people go about solving problems, with a group dimension added (Atherton 2005). It was developed in the 1940s by Revans, a physicist who first developed it from his experience of team working and employed it as a tool in the coal industry to improve production (Smith & O'Neil 2003). He later went on to use action learning with hospital managers in the early 1970s and whilst it has proved popular in management education as an approach to problem-based learning, it also has a clear attraction as a learning tool in health-care organisations. It has been adopted as a means to achieving organisational goals as well as identifying problems and testing and adopting solutions. Put simply, it is an approach to problem-based learning, or solving problems in groups, where the learning is through experience 'by doing', where the task environment is a classroom and the task is the vehicle for learning (Smith & O'Neil 2003). It has been used in health care as a tool for implementing research evidence in primary care (Foy *et al.* 2002) by academic institutions to support practice-based learning (O'Hara *et al.* 1997; Koo 1999), and in medical quality management to support leadership in health services. It is a concept that appears to work well where there is an identified problem or learning need that can be addressed through reflection, questioning and the implementation of group-generated ideas.

In this sense, action learning is a process that uses a peer group or set to generate action plans and to generate learning from reflection on practice (Beaty *et al.* 1997). O'Hara *et al.* (1997) state that

> 'at its best an action learning set is a learning community where members want one another to succeed and where they support and challenge one another's ideas and actions from their assessment of what will be most helpful at any particular moment.'

Since Revans' original work to develop action learning, there have been multiple variations of the concept, but all share the elements of real people resolving real problems in real time and learning while doing so (Marquardt 2004). It appears to work best where there is an action-based approach to developing options and plans to resolving practice issues in a community (or action learning set) where a group is faced with problems and is capable of using a questioning approach to identifying and testing potential solutions to them.

Engaging a group in action learning over time has been successful in many areas, although there is limited evidence that action learning can support CPD in clear practice terms. However, what seems to be a common theme throughout the literature on action learning is that it is both a useful and appropriate vehicle for professional and personal development. The opportunity for reflection on experience, learning from that reflection and planning for action fit well with the notion of professional autonomy and personal responsibility for development (Beaty *et al.* 1997). Certainly in relation to non-medical prescribing, one would anticipate that a group of set members, such as non-medical prescribers, would be sufficiently experienced to value the scrutiny and support of peers in a learning environment. In this respect, a questioning and open approach to professional development in relation to the prescribing role is welcome, in particular, where the practitioner is striving for a level of practice beyond basic competence.

Who will benefit from action learning?

O'Hara *et al.* (1997) use their extensive experience in facilitating action learning to identify the kinds of people who benefit most from action learning and indeed who will be least likely to benefit. Given that an essential element of action learning is the action, planned or speculated as an outcome from learning, then the people most likely to be able to pursue action as a result of group interaction are those who have autonomy and are therefore in a position to influence practice at their own level, at least. This implies that a member of an action learning set should be in a position of some authority. Whilst action learning was developed primarily as a management tool, however, this does not necessarily mean that those who do not hold management positions are inappropriate members of a set. What it requires though, is that one has sufficient authority in one's own practice area and that one can make decisions about, for example, how to develop, change or drive forward practice.

Whilst it is difficult to learn through action learning if one does not hold a position of authority, however, it is also difficult if you are not willing to take action (O'Hara et al. 1997). This may simply be related to learning styles, and for those who have learned teacher dependence, it may take significant time to develop the skills to influence practice from the learning taking place within the set. If one is simply looking for teacher-centred approaches to development, then action learning may be a poor choice. In any event, the members of an action learning set need to have some investment in finding a solution to a problem or problems (Atherton 2005), and in this context, problems that occur in everyday practice. A particular skill that forms one of the absolute prerequisites for action learning is reflection.

Reflection as both skill and process has for some time underpinned elements of learning for many of the health professions, although to varying degrees. Whilst the set promotes reflection, if its members are not prepared to reflect, then they will derive little benefit from that part of the learning process. O'Hara et al. (1997) use their experience to note the importance of set members wanting to use action learning and one must certainly acknowledge that a reflective, and sometimes intense process of learning, is not the approach to learning that some individuals want. If one comes to the action learning approach with the intention of understanding it and making it work, however, it can be a powerful learning tool – it 'does not seem to work well for people who are talked into it'. Importantly, it is for those who are looking for learning that it connects directly with something they are doing. Within health care one has to consider the motivation and commitment of individuals to action learning, and whether this is a priority for them. Our experience is that whilst many might feel they will benefit from action learning as part of a group of professionals from varied specialities in the broader sense of approaches to prescribing practice and organisational influences on it, there are equally those who do not feel they have any learning to gain from those out with their very focused sphere of practice and would prefer to see action learning centred entirely on their own speciality.

It must be argued that on the basis of O'Hara *et al.*'s (1997) experience, the simple pre-requisite for entry to non-medical prescribing training that practitioners are experienced in their field, is sufficient to almost guarantee a set of mature adults who are willing to embrace change and practice development on the basis of reflection and action, although this may not necessarily be the case. In our experience, learning from these approaches, to a high degree in health services, depends on authority. Whilst O'Hara *et al.* acknowledge that this is the case; within health services there are organisational rules and hierarchies that can either support or hinder the success of any development that might come from action learning.

What kind of organisation makes action learning a success?

Most health-care organisations are complex, but in the context of non-medical prescribing, we are dealing firstly with people. These are our patients, colleagues, peers, senior management, medical colleagues and other professional groups. Many of us additionally work closely with external agencies. As such, we are bound by rules and governance in relation to practice and process and importantly, confidentiality. Creating change within an organisation resistant to it is difficult, and change requires organisational support. Lawson *et al.* (1997) clearly support this observation by asserting the view that an organisation that welcomes change and evolution of practice is central to the support of action learning. Equally important is the organisation that encourages the generation and testing of ideas, and particularly, one that supports autonomy. Line manager support is important and therefore the culture of the organisation should be one that encourages and values action learning. The difficulty with health-care organisations in the twenty-first century, however, is that many are so large that organisational sub-culture can exist even within departments or divisions, particularly in large acute or Primary Care Trusts. What might be an exceptionally supportive environment for action learning in one area may be particularly difficult in another, and so whether action learning will work well in a particular area is frequently dependent on departmental personalities and management styles. In this respect, it is imperative that any organisational non-medical prescribing policy lends clear support to a variety of approaches to CPD.

Putting action learning into practice

Atherton (2005) provides a very simple and practical guide to action learning. The ideal size of the set is four to six members, who meet as a closed group for an indeterminate period that might stretch to several months. Members take turns in presenting an update on their work, and then being questioned by other group members, who act as consultants or mentors to each other. The nature of questioning is important, and action learning theorists will expand on the science of questioning. In essence, however, questioning should be open and inquisitive rather than adversarial. It is intended to promote reflection and planning for action in order to devise an action plan, which the member fulfils outside the group, for further discussion at a future meeting.

The set advisor, or facilitator, will be experienced in action learning and will start by establishing ground rules, modelling the question process and pointing members in the direction of potential resources. As the set members grow in confidence, the facilitator will take a smaller part in the activity of the group, and as a successful set matures, the group members may take on the role of a facilitator (McGill & Beaty 2001).

Facilitation

Given the need for organisational commitment and the potential for organisational learning from the experience of group members, it is useful to speculate as to whether the set advisor or facilitator should be a senior member of a health-care organisation, for example, a senior manager or non-medical prescribing lead. Jones *et al*. (2005) describe a project that engaged their early non-medical prescribers in action learning, which was initiated by an organisational need to provide CPD for a small group of prescribers. Agreement was reached that action learning was a useful approach to this and six set meetings, with four members were arranged. These were facilitated by a deputy director of nursing and had a clear agenda for the set members – to network with colleagues, give and receive information, share practice and receive supervision. Jones *et al*. (2005) describe a process of learning that identified learning needs common to all prescribers, for example, obtaining consent, devising an audit trail of prescriptions, support and role modelling and access to advice and literature for potential new prescribers.

They set out clear benefits of the learning to set members that were achieved as a result of the involvement of deputy directors of nursing as facilitators, an involvement that demonstrated clear corporate support as well as a developing understanding of practical issues involved in non-medical prescribing, for the directors themselves to feed back to the organisation. For prescribers, to have the reassurance that senior organisational representatives were informed about current practice, and had the opportunity to develop an understanding of their evolving practice context, was an important factor. From the organisational perspective, the benefit of involving senior management was noted in terms of its impact on 'corporate knowledge about nurse prescribing which resulted in corporate governance issues which were subsequently actioned by set members themselves' (Jones *et al.* 2005).

However, in deciding, whether a senior member of an organisational management team should be involved in facilitating an action learning set, one should consider professional issues such as confidentiality, as well as whether the set members feel confident and comfortable that their discussions are clearly confidential and take place where they feel 'safe' in terms of expressing views or discussing difficulties in practice. Largely, this is an issue for both the set and the organisation to deal with. Whilst there is clear potential for organisational benefit in involving senior managers, it is also possible that this could be gained by using a facilitator with a practice and/or educational, rather than managerial, background to help address practice issues.

Practical experience – organisational action learning

The value of action learning, and in particular, learning from one's own and others' experience, is exceptional. However, in practical terms, getting even a committed action learning set together is difficult. With a group of over 70 non-medical prescribers in a single organisation, even getting a small number together can be a logistical nightmare. Whilst this is the case, our experience has been that with dates set far enough in advance, barring last-minute clinical priorities, a small cross-speciality, multi-professional group has developed within that far larger number. Outside of this, there is a commitment to hold directorate level, rather than organisational level, groups. Where disparate groups for action learning develop, for example, within specialities, it is important that there continues to be a forum that monitors or develops learning and CPD activity across the organisation. In smaller organisations with less diverse working patterns, it is more realistic to maintain a constant set who meet regularly, with protected time.

Whichever way sets are generated, by organisational or directorate level initiation, an important element is the setting of ground rules. These should address areas of importance, such as the course that meetings should follow and the rules around confidentiality and questioning; set members should agree on the role of the facilitator as well as the members from the outset.

In each group, set members might present particular issues that have arisen in practice or case studies (see Section Three, Appendix 6:2 for an example of case study presentation), and true to the ethos of action learning, other set members will spend time questioning and discussing the issues that arise. For example, issues that have arisen include those around organisational policy, prescribing for children, mandatory CPD and how we address the issue of some managers in the organisation attempting to restrict prescribing to an agreed list of drugs, rather than a recognised Trust-wide formulary (see Box 6.1 for an example of subjects for action learning and learning sets). Areas that group members have explored and helped others to learn have been in negotiating their role as a prescriber or using the influence of the organisation to support prescribing in respect to national prescribing guidance, rather than in relation to local 'rules' generated by those who do not have a clear understanding of policy guidance and the account-ability of non-medical prescribers. We have addressed issues that arise from incorporating prescribing into individuals' job descriptions and informed the development of other approaches to CPD around the organisation by maintaining a two-way communication with senior members of the organisational management team. Some of the issues start out as being problematic for a single set member, but by addressing them early on in the development of non-medical prescribing, we have headed off potentially greater issues for a larger number of prescribers.

Box 6.1 Examples of subjects arising in action learning and learning sets

- Input to organisational non-medical prescribing policy
- Communication pathways for new information and policies that affect non-medical prescribers
- Dissemination of new information, for example, new outpatient pre-scribing policy, medicines management policy or updated antibiotic prescribing policy
- Discussion and input into consultations and responses (for example Medicines and Health-care products Regulatory Agency (MHRA) con-sultations on expanding non-medical prescribing to new professional groups)
- Update on cross-organisational services that support prescribing prac-tice, for example, diabetes management and antibiotic prescribing
- Evaluation of the effects of non-medical prescribing services on the patient pathway, for example, diabetes, chest pain, acute pain and total parenteral nutrition (TPN) services.

There are clear elements of learning from the sets that have two dis-tinct focuses. Firstly, individual learning for those involved, by 'talking through' issues with others in a similar position and who understand the context of their work. Secondly, learning for the organisation, and this is as important. From the perspective of individual learning about practice, each meeting holds a clear opportunity, with individual members of the wider group asked periodically to discuss general areas of patient management that might impact on a wider group of prescribers, for example, pain control, the development of Trust policy for antibiotic use or outpatient prescribing and diabetes updates. In organisational terms, we are often getting to grips with how and where non-medical prescribing is effective and the meetings therefore provide an excellent opportunity for organisational questions or feedback to be raised. Issues that have arisen, ranging from individuals with poor understanding of legislation attempting to limit the development of non-medical prescribing, to addressing how we go about monitoring non-medical prescribing activity, have been addressed. Audit forms an important part of the work of an action learning group or learning set and supports non-medical prescribers in developing the organisation' awareness of achievements of non-medical prescribers (see Section Three, Appendix 6:2, which offers a Department of Health example relating to evaluating the implementation of non-medical prescribing in delivering service improvements). Importantly, action learning has input to the development of the non-medical prescribing policy and therefore has allowed non-medical prescribers to have a direct organisational impact. There has also been significant cross-speciality learning through identified learning needs such as critical appraisal of research evidence and managing pharmaceutical company representation, as well as the opportunity to update in relation to non-medical prescribing developments regionally and nationally and the opportunity to contribute to the organisational response to national consultations.

Practical experience – learning sets in a single speciality

Apart from those benefits gained through organisational learning, many non-medical prescribers are looking for specific learning, in relation to their own speciality, and many want 'updates' provided for them whilst discussing practice issues relating to prescribing. In this sense, a set operating at directorate level, with updates, for example, in relation to pharmacology in a narrow field, are not focused only around action learning, but can still be thought of as 'learning sets'. Discrete, multi-professional teams of non-medical prescribers working in a single speciality can plan to come together as frequently as they would like to discuss developments in their field, for example, diabetes specialists, cardiac nurse and pharmacist specialists, pain control nurses, children's nurses and multi-professional groups working in oncology with responsibility for prescribing. Involving medical teams in discussions at this level in particular also serves to raise the profile of non-medical prescribing and can widen an extremely important medical support network. In fact, apart from continuing supervisory relationships with medical staff, this is perhaps one of the best opportunities in our experience to develop a non-medical prescribing support network amongst a wide range of medical staff.

Additional benefits of action learning and learning sets

Whether non-medical prescribers are coming together as a multi-professional group or as a single group of professionals, whether at an organisational level or at the level of a single speciality, the opportunity to come together and discuss issues is a valuable support mechanism. It offers the opportunity to discuss the benefits to the organisation of non-medical prescribing and indeed we have amassed a huge amount of data that support its implementation in a wide range of settings. For example, the use of a simple audit tool (Figure 6.1) for each prescriber allows us to audit the effects of prescribing by nurses, pharmacists and allied health professionals on the achievement of organisational goals. These range from improving accessibility to time-dependent treatment for patients, reducing time spent for patients waiting for junior medical staff to write prescriptions for medications 'to take out' (TTO) and indeed expediting the process of patient admission, access to appropriate and timely treatment and reducing length of hospital stay. Using learning sets to present Trust or directorate-wide data offers significant positive reinforcement and an opportunity to discuss what further developments across the patient pathway might further achieve organisational goals.

Conclusion

Action learning, particularly at an organisational level, is valuable to both individual practitioners and to the organisation, provided that the set members hold the organisational authority necessary to develop or influence practice and have organisational support. Organisational learning is also an important aspect of action learning and there should be clear routes for set members to feed back perceived organisational influences on prescribing practice. At a directorate or practice level, it can be an excellent vehicle for extending learning beyond principles of practice into a speciality as well as for providing an exceptional cross-professional support system. Action learning does not suit every organisation or indeed every individual, but has certainly demonstrated its value as a practice-focused approach to CPD.

Date	Patient Identifier/ Name & Hospital No	Inpatient / Outpatient	Diagnosis	Medication(s) prescribed	Rationale for decision to prescribe / not prescribe

Name:

Cinical area:

Figure 6.1   Audit/data collection sheet – non-medical prescribing.

Key learning points

- Action learning is a tried and tested method of approaching learning in health care, though till date it has largely been used as a management development tool.
- Action learning can be a useful approach to CPD for non-medical prescribers and can be offered either at an organisational or at a speciality level.
- Action learning can provide a forum for developing understanding of the context of prescribing both for the organisation and for individual prescribers.
- A learning set can be a valuable organisational resource for gathering audit data in order to demonstrate the effectiveness and impact of non-medical prescribing.
- Learning sets can be a useful forum for maintaining and developing inter-professional learning.

Key resources in Section Three

- Department of Health 'Making the Connections' document, highlighting the organisational benefits of non-medical prescribing
- Example case study discussed at an action learning set
- Example Medicines Information Leaflets and examples of good practice in disseminating prescribing guidance in acute care.

References

Atherton, J. S. (2005) *Teaching and Learning: Action Learning* [On-line] UK. Available at: http://www.learningandteaching.info/teaching/action_learning.htm [Accessed: 6 June 2008].

Beaty, L., Lawson, J., Bourner, T. and O'Hara, S. (1997) Action learning comes of age – part 3: action learning for what? *Education and Training* 39(5): 184–188.

Bourner, T. (1996) cited in Koo L.C. (1999) Learning action learning. *Journal of Workplace Learning* 11(3): 89–94.

Foy, R., Tidy, N. and Hollis, S. (2002) Inter-professional learning in primary care: lessons form an action learning programme. *British Journal of Clinical Governance* 7(1): 40–44.

Jones, K., Brown, W., Bunker, J., Heywood, S., Howard, D. and Van Tromp, J. (2005) Action learning to provide continuing professional development. *Nurse Prescribing* 3(4): 156–158.

Koo, L. (1999) Learning action learning. *Journal of Workplace Learning* 11(3): 89.

Lawson, J., Beaty, L., Bourner, T. and O'Hara, S. (1997) Action learning comes of age – part 4. *Education and Training* 39(6): 225–229.

Marquardt, M. (2004) Harnessing the power of action learning. *Training and Development* 58(6): 26–32.

McGill, I. and Beaty, L. (2001) *Action Learning. A Guide for Professional, Management and Educational Development*, 2nd edition. London, Kogan Page.

O'Hara, S., Beaty, L., Lawson, J. and Bourner, T. (1997) Action learning comes of age – part 2: action learning for whom? *Education and Training* 39(2): 91–95.

Smith, P. and O'Neil, J. (2003) A review of action learning literature 1994–2000: part 1 – bibliography and comments. *Journal of Workplace Learning* 15(2): 63–69.

7 Keeping Up to Date with Pharmacology

Nicola Stoner

Introduction

This chapter will emphasise the importance of up to date pharmacological knowledge to remain competent as a non-medical prescriber. In order to put this into context, a summary will be provided of what is currently known about the pharmacological knowledge of qualified non-medical prescribers and how this may impact on prescribing practice.

Some key elements of basic pharmacological principles will be presented. This may provide helpful revision for continuing professional development (CPD) purposes either for the individual or for adaptation for training purposes by the employing organisation. The chapter will also include some pharmacology teaching and learning exercises, which we have used within our CPD prescribing workshops. The chapter will also be supported within the resources section (Appendix 7) with a number of online sources, which can be accessed in order to keep up to date with pharmacology.

Background and the need to keep up to date with pharmacology

Pharmacology explains how drugs act inside a patient to produce its effects. Clinical pharmacology is the science of drugs and their clinical use. The pharmacological effect of a drug can be monitored by its clinical effect or by measuring its concentration in the body. The pharmacology of drugs has several key elements, which are briefly described later in this chapter.

Knowledge of the pharmacology of drugs is essential to non-medical prescribers in order to prescribe the correct medication at the right dose, via the right route and frequency of administration for the patient to achieve the desired therapeutic response with minimum toxicity (BMJ 2007a, 2007b).

The pharmacology of the drugs being prescribed underpins all of this, so it is essential that the individual maintains their competence in, and understanding of, pharmacology (NPC 2001, 2003a, 2003b, 2004, NMC 2006). Non-medical prescribers must understand the potential of undesired effects such as adverse drug reactions, drug interactions, allergies and side effects. They must be aware of how to avoid or minimise these unwanted effects and how to manage them should they occur. They must also have an appreciation of the misuse potential of drugs.

It is essential that non-medical prescribers have current knowledge relating to the products they prescribe, for example, doses, formulations, pack sizes, storage conditions and costs. They also need to be confident in their knowledge of all the drugs they prescribe so that they are able to answer questions from patients to ensure that patients are fully informed partners in their treatments to improve compliance and concordance.

Research is ongoing to find better and more effective drugs and drug targets for all medical conditions. New drugs that work in different ways are always coming into the market. Non-medical prescribers need to know how to acquire and deal with new information about new or existing drugs.

It is implicit that non-medical prescribers combine their knowledge of pharmacology with principles of evidence-based practice as applied to prescribing. The application of these principles for CPD purposes are discussed in Chapter 9 of this book.

Pharmacology education for non-medical prescribers

The curriculum for non-medical prescribing courses within the United Kingdom was outlined by the Department of Health and the Nursing and Midwifery Council (2004, 2006). This specifies the indicative teaching and learning content and this includes clinical pharmacology including the effects of co-morbidity. Non-medical prescribing students are typically taught general principles such as pharmacokinetics, pharmacodynamics and adverse drug reactions.

This can be challenging for providers of the training who are charged with delivering the course over a 26-day teaching period and also has to include consultation, decision making and therapy, including referral, influences on and psychology of prescribing; prescribing in a team context; evidence-based practice and clinical governance in relation to prescribing, legal, policy and ethical concepts, professional accountability and responsibility and prescribing within a public health context.

Lymn *et al.* (2008) have highlighted that the shift away from biological sciences to a social science model of nursing education means that many qualified nurses who embark on a prescribing course can have very limited pre-exposure to basic biological concepts, which are crucial to the understanding of elementary pharmacology principles. Courtenay and Latter (2003) and Banning (2004) have also highlighted the importance of bio-sciences within nurse education. The outcome of the developments within non-medical prescribing have recognised the need for nurses to have a sound understanding of pharmacology; Banning also suggests the importance of the understanding of science, pathophysiology, applied pharmacology and diagnostics as a component of nurse pre-registration training in order to prepare for a future prescribing role.

Furthermore, Offredy *et al.* (2007) and Sodha *et al.* (2002) have found that some nurses who had undertaken a prescribing course did not possess a sufficient depth of knowledge of pharmacology in order to make them feel confident or competent within their prescribing role. This can lead to a tendency to not fully utilise prescribing skills and responsibilities and, therefore, develop ongoing competence and mastery.

In relation to CPD for prescribers, this is very important because it suggests that there is a need to ensure continuing development of pharmacological knowledge. For the employing organisation, this may involve assessment of pharmacological knowledge in order to determine the limits of a prescribing role and plan for future training and development. The use of prescribing case studies as suggested by Offredy *et al.* (2007) in order to facilitate this will be discussed later in the chapter.

Key elements of pharmacology

Pharmacokinetics

Pharmacokinetics describes what happens to the drug while it is in the body. It forms the basis of drug dosing, frequency of administration, dose alterations required in certain clinical conditions, and the mechanism of some drug interactions. Pharmacokinetics involves the body systems for handling the drug, as described below (Thomson 2004a).

Absorption

In order for a drug to get to its target in the body it needs to be absorbed. The oral route of administration is the most convenient, but can be the most challenging. Drugs administered orally have to be stable in acid, and absorbed through the walls of the gastrointestinal tract. Some patient characteristics can affect absorption, for example, the rate of gastric emptying, the amount of acid produced in the stomach, or any disorders of the gastrointestinal tract (McGavock 2001a; Thomson 2004a).

Drugs are manufactured using several strategies to ensure absorption. For example, the drug's physical and chemical properties may need to be changed, the formulation adapted or the drug administered by a different route. Drugs can be formulated in certain ways to improve their absorption, such as in a sustained release, enteric coated or liquid formulation. Alternative routes of drug administration include oral, rectal, and nasogastric; subcutaneous, intra-dermal, intramuscular or intravenous injection; inhalation, sublingual, buccal, topical, or trans-dermal. There are advantages and disadvantages of all of these routes (McGavock 2001a; Thomson 2004a).

Drugs given orally often need to be given in higher doses than those given intravenously. Oral drugs are often less 'bioavailable' as less of the drug is available in the body once it has gone through the pharmacokinetic steps. Intravenous drug administration ensures that they are 100% bioavailable (McGavock 2001a; Thomson 2004a).

Distribution

Once a drug has been absorbed into the body, it is transported around the body via the blood stream. The concentration of a drug in any specific tissue depends on its physical and chemical properties, how soluble it is in fat or water, whether it crosses the blood–brain barrier and the blood flow to that tissue (McGavock 2001b; Thomson 2004a). The volume of distributions gives a measure of the amount of drug in the blood stream after it has been absorbed and can be used to calculate the concentration of a particular dose in the blood stream using the calculation seen in Box 7.1.

Box 7.1 The volume of distribution

$$D/V = C$$

V = volume of distribution
D = dose
C = concentration of the drug in the blood stream

Protein binding of a drug affects its distribution. Drugs that stay in the blood stream because they bind to plasma proteins or are water soluble have a small volume of distribution. Those that are distributed throughout the body with very little remaining in the blood stream or are fat soluble have a large volume of distribution. Water-soluble drugs can collect in 'third space' fluid collections as in patients with extensive oedema, ascites or pleural effusions. Fat-soluble drugs may collect in the fat of obese patients (McGavock 2001b; Thomson 2004a).

Elimination and metabolism

Drugs are eliminated from the body in a variety of ways. They can be eliminated via the kidneys, liver, breast milk, bile, sweat or from a person's breath (Thomson 2004a).

Renal elimination

Elimination via the kidney depends on the blood flow to the kidney, how well the kidneys are working (the glomerular filtration rate) and whether a drug is actively secreted from or passively reabsorbed back into the tubule. Patients with renal failure or dysfunction, older patients or neonates may require a dose reduction for renally eliminated drugs (McGavock 2001c; Thomson 2004a).

Liver metabolism

Elimination of drugs via the liver depends on the blood flow to the liver and enzyme activity in the liver. Liver enzymes chemically alter or metabolise drugs to make them inactive, more active, or equally active to the original drug. Drugs that are metabolised in the liver are usually eliminated via the kidney as they become more water soluble. There are some factors that may alter elimination via the liver. For example, older patients tend to have a poorer blood flow to the liver, and neonates have low liver enzyme activity. If patients have extensive liver damage, this may affect their ability to metabolise a drug that is normally metabolised in the liver (McGavock 2001d; Thomson 2004a,b).

Some drugs affect the liver enzymes by either inducing them to break down drugs faster or by inhibiting them so that drugs are broken down more slowly. If a drug induces liver enzymes, then a larger dose of the affected drug is required to get the same clinical effect. If the drug is broken down more slowly because of liver enzymes being inhibited, then a smaller dose of the affected drug would be needed to get the same clinical effect (McGavock 2001d; Thomson 2004a,b). Table 7.1 shows examples of drugs that induce and inhibit liver enzymes.

Table 7.1 Examples of drugs that induce or inhibit liver enzymes.

Drugs that induce liver enzymes	Drugs that inhibit liver enzymes
Alcohol	Amiodarone
Carbamazepine	Calcium channel blockers
Griseofulvin	Cimetidine
Phenytoin	Ciprofloxacin
Phenobarbitone	Erythromycin
Rifampicin	Fluconazole
	Omeprazole
	Oral contraceptives
	Omeprazole

Entero-hepatic circulation

Entero-hepatic circulation can occur for some drugs. This means that the drug is excreted from the liver to the bile. As the drug enters the duodenum, it is de-conjugated and may be reabsorbed. The drug then goes through the same route again. Any drug that is circulated in this way stays in the body for longer, as the process prolongs the half-life of the drug. Examples of drugs that are affected by entero-hepatic circulation include diazepam and oestrogen. For example, diazepam is conjugated in the liver and some of the resulting diazepam glucuronide is excreted into the bile and then to the intestine, where the glucuronide bond is de-conjugated by intestinal enzymes. The free diazepam is then reabsorbed and the cycle starts again. Patients on the oral contraceptive pill must be warned to use additional precautions if they have diarrhoea from any cause, as diarrhoea will reduce the time of entero-hepatic circulation, thus reducing plasma oestrogen levels and resulting in the failure of the oral contraceptive (McGavock 2001d).

First-pass effect

Oral drugs that are absorbed from the gastrointestinal tract are sometimes carried to the liver via the hepatic portal vein. Drugs that are carried through this route can sometimes be partially or completely metabolised by the liver before they reach the blood stream and the drug's ultimate target. This is called the *first-pass metabolism*, and means that the quantity of drug available in the body is reduced. Sometimes drugs have to be administered by alternative routes to avoid this first-pass effect, for example, intravenously or sublingually. For example, the first-pass effect inactivates drugs such as lignocaine and glyceryl trinitrate (McGavock 2001d).

Therapeutic drug monitoring

The dosing interval of a drug is determined by its half-life. The half-life is the time taken for the concentration of a drug in the blood to fall by half of its original value. The aim is to ensure that the drug remains in the body at a steady level or concentration, avoiding too large a peak (maximum drug level) or too low a trough (ineffective drug level) (Thomson 2004a).

Some drugs have a narrow therapeutic index. That means that there is a small difference between plasma levels for an ineffective dose and a toxic dose. Examples of drugs with a narrow therapeutic index include digoxin, gentamicin, carbamazepine, phenytoin, lithium and theophylline. Plasma concentrations of these drugs often have to be monitored.

Some drugs produce variable plasma concentrations in different people, for example, warfarin, and the levels of the drug in the system, or the therapeutic response to them, has to be monitored. The reasons for this could be the individual differences in absorption, metabolism, distribution and elimination. Patients with gastrointestinal, hepatic, renal or cardiovascular disease may have different plasma levels for the same dose. Drug interactions and poor compliance will also affect drug levels.

Loading dose

For some drugs, when initiating treatment, it is necessary to give an initial loading dose to ensure that there is an adequate concentration of the drug in the body to have an effect immediately, and a well-known example of this is digoxin. Once the target plasma concentration is achieved, a maintenance dose needs to be administered (Thomson 2004a).

Pharmacodynamics

Pharmacodynamics describes what drugs do to the body and how. The way the drug works is usually dependent on the chemical composition of the drug. Drugs work in one of several ways as described below.

Drugs acting on receptors

Some drugs work by acting on specific proteins called *receptors*, which can either be on cell membranes or inside the cells. The receptor theory is known as the *lock and key concept*. The drug (key) is designed to fit into the receptor (lock) in order to exert its action. The structure and shape of a drug defines its drug–receptor interaction. When a drug binds to a receptor, this leads to a series of pathways that culminate in the biological effect of the drug (McGavock 2001e, 2001f, 2002a).

Drugs can block receptors and act as antagonists to inhibit a natural substance from binding with the receptor. Antagonists can work by being competitive or non-competitive. Alternatively, drugs can bind to the receptor in order to stimulate the receptor, acting as an agonist. Agonists usually behave like the natural molecule that normally binds with that receptor. Side effects can occur because drugs are not specific to certain receptors or because they also act on other areas of the body (McGavock 2001e, 2001f, 2002a).

Enzyme inhibition

Drugs can block the action of specific enzymes in order to exert their effect. Side effects occur when the enzymes blocked are found both in the desired target and elsewhere in the body (McGavock 2001e, 2001f, 2002a).

Drugs affecting cell transport

Drugs can affect cellular transport mechanisms in order to exert their effect. For example, calcium channel blockers block ion channels in the cell membrane of the vascular smooth muscle, and so interfere with the movement of ions across cell membranes. Ion channels are like gates that open and close to let substances through (McGavock 2001e, 2001f, 2002a).

Non-specific actions

Some drugs have non-specific actions. For example, antacids such as aluminium hydroxide will neutralise acid in the stomach, or emollients will moisturise the skin (McGavock 2001e, 2001f, 2002a).

Drug action on invading organisms

Antimicrobial drugs work in several different ways, depending on the individual drug groups. For example, beta-lactam antibiotics such as penicillin inhibit the synthesis of the bacterial cell wall (McGavock 2002b). Antibiotics must be prescribed according to local guidelines, which represent local resistance patterns, to ensure appropriate pre-scribing. Inappropriate antibiotic prescribing can lead to antibiotic resistance and the emergence of super-bugs.

Pharmacogenetics

There can be genetic factors involved in the biotransformation of some drugs. This can mean that there is a variation in the pharmacokinetics and pharmacodynamics of a drug in an individual, family or race. This is termed *pharmacogenetics*. Genetic screening is likely to be undertaken in the future to tailor drug treatments to individual patients so that such genetic differences in drug absorption, metabolism, and elimination can be taken into account. This should help to minimise toxicity or the use of ineffective treatments in some patients (Thomson 2004b).

Drug interactions

Drug interactions can be divided into pharmacokinetic and pharmaco-dynamic drug interactions. Pharmacodynamic interactions occur when drugs have similar or antagonistic pharmacological effects or side effects. These may be due to competition at receptor sites or the action of drugs on the same physiological system. Pharmacokinetic interactions occur when one drug alters the absorption, distribution, metabolism or excretion of another, thus increasing or reducing the amount of drug available to produce its pharmacological effects. Drug interactions can be harmful or beneficial. Some are clinically significant and some are not (McGavock 2002c; Thomson 2004b).

Important drug interactions to consider are those with drugs with a narrow therapeutic index, drugs that inhibit or induce enzymes, drugs with known pharmacodynamic effects or those with susceptible pharmacokinetics, like oral contraceptives or oral hypoglycaemics.

A drug's volume of distribution can also affect its interactions. For example, drugs with a low volume of distribution may interact with drugs affecting plasma proteins. Drugs with a high volume of distribution may need to have their doses reduced if there is impairment of the circulation, for example, in congestive cardiac failure (McGavock 2002c; Thomson 2004b).

Adverse drug reactions

Adverse drug reactions are harmful or unpleasant effects of drugs that occur at doses that are intended for prophylaxis, diagnosis or treat-ment. They necessitate drugs to be withdrawn or to have their dose reduced. Adverse drug events are the most common cause of iatro-genic injury in hospital patients. There are two types of adverse drug reactions – predictable (type A) and unpredictable (type B). Type A reactions are common, dose-related side effects due to an excessive pharmacological effect. Type B reactions are infrequent and include allergic and idiosyncratic reactions or genetically determined effects (McGavock 2002d).

Adverse drug reactions must be reported on a yellow card, which is found at the back of the British National Formulary (BNF). When assessing whether a patient may have had an adverse drug reaction, consideration needs to be given to the patient's susceptibility, possible drug interactions, the timing of starting and stopping the drug or doses being changed in relation to the symptoms, and the possibility of another medical condition causing the symptoms (McGavock 2002d).

It is essential to minimise the risk of adverse events when prescribing. These can be minimised by always including a detailed drug history in any consultation, only using a drug when there is clear indication to do so, stopping drugs that are no longer necessary, and checking the dose and response especially in young, older, pregnant or breastfeeding patients and those with renal, hepatic, or cardiac disease (McGavock 2002d, 2002e; Thomson 2004b).

Pharmacology teaching and learning exercises

Lymn *et al.* (2008) have highlighted the fact that teaching basic pharmacological principles can be a 'dry business'. It is therefore important to consider creative ways in which to facilitate the understanding of the learner. As we have discussed already, there are limits within prescribing courses about the amount of pharmacology that can be delivered and some non-medical prescribers do not feel confident about their pharmacological knowledge. The following section contains a selection of teaching and learning exercises, which may be adapted for CPD learning needs. We have included some multiple choice questions, which we have used both in our prescribing courses and in assessing knowledge within the CPD prescribing workshops that we run.

Offredy *et al.* (2007) used prescribing case histories or exercises to encourage the use of the BNF in order to assess pharmacological knowledge of a group of nurse prescribers. We have included a selection of BNF exercises that will encourage the learner to apply pharmacological principles. We have also used these exercises within the CPD prescribing workshops that we run. Alternatively, prescribers can present case histories from their own area of clinical prescribing practice.

We have included an example of a drug proforma as seen in Figure 7.1. Within the prescribing courses that we run we encourage the students to build their own personal formularies and suggest that this is an

Drug Proforma	
Pharmacological class	
Mechanism of action Pharmacokinetics Pharmacodynamics	
Preparations	
Indications	
Side-effects	
Cautions	
Contraindications	
Side-effects	

Figure 7.1   Example drug profile proforma.

activity to be continued within CPD; the proforma can be used for individual reflection or as a basis of discussion within workshops or action learning groups as discussed in Chapters 4 and 6.

Pharmacology self-test

Multiple choice questions
1. Most antagonists work by competition, thus the effect of competitive antagonists can be overcome by increasing the amount of agonist. True OR False?
2. Which of the following statements is inaccurate?
   (a) Ligands and receptors chemically bind with a reversible chemical bond.

    (b)   Chemical bonds between ligands and receptors cause structural change in the receptor, which results in transduction leading to alteration of cell function.

    (c)   The transducer site cannot be targeted for chemical modification by drugs.

    (d)   Transduction describes intermediate processes between formation of the drug receptor complex and the effect.

3.   A drug allergy

    (a)   Occurs when too much drug has accumulated in an individual

    (b)   Occurs when the body sees the drug as an antigen and an immune response is established against the drug

    (c)   Occurs in a predictable manner as a desirable response to a drug

    (d)   Is a Type E adverse drug reaction

4.   Adverse drug reactions are responses to administered drugs which

    (a)   Are not noxious

    (b)   Are intended

    (c)   Occur at doses higher than recommended doses

    (d)   Are responsible for a significant number of hospital admissions

5.   Which of the following would you NOT report using the yellow card?

    (a)   A suspected minor side effect to an existing drug

    (b)   A suspected minor side effect to a black triangle drug

    (c)   A suspected serious side effect to a black triangle drug

    (d)   A suspected minor side effect to a herbal remedy

6.   Under the yellow card reporting system which of the following would NOT be classified as a reportable ADR?

    (a)   A 40 year-old woman who died in hospital after an allergic reaction to a vaccine

    (b)   A 68 year-old man with prolonged diarrhoea after taking a herbal tonic

    (c)   A 19 year-old who has slept badly for one night after taking pseudoephedrine tablets for nasal decongestion

    (d)   A 42 year-old who was admitted to hospital with a reaction to an IUD fitted from a new batch of supplies

7.   A 'Type E' adverse drug reaction to an administered drug relates to

    (a)   Adverse reactions that result from continuous administration of a drug

    (b)   Adverse drug reactions resulting from discontinuation of drug therapy

    (c)   Adverse reactions that are bizarre and non-dose related

    (d)   Adverse drug reactions which occur after a long delay

8.   The most reliable indicator or combination of indicators for paediatric calculation is/are

    (a)   Height and body weight

    (b)   Body surface area

    (c)   Sex and race

    (d)   Age and sex

9.   Ibuprofen is a useful

    (a)   CNS stimulant

    (b)   Antidepressant

      (c)   Urosacic acid

      (d)   Non-steroidal anti inflammatory agent (NSAID)

10. A two year-old child has contracted an infection and antibiotic therapy is indicated. Based on this information alone, according to the BNF which of the following should NOT be prescribed?

      (a)   Penicillin

      (b)   Erythromycin

      (c)   Tetracycline

      (d)   Amoxycillin

11. Which one of the following statements is incorrect?

      (a)   Continuous blockade of receptors by an antagonist on long-term use results in upregulation of receptors to the antagonist that could lead to withdrawal effects on sudden cessation of therapy.

      (b)   Continuous stimulation of receptors by an agonist on long-term use leads to down-regulation of receptors to the agonist that could lead to tolerance.

      (c)   Upregulation of receptors indicates that receptors have decreased numbers or sensitivity and this means increasing doses of the agonist is required to obtain the same effect.

      (d)   Down-regulation of receptors indicates that receptors have decreased in numbers or sensitivity and this means increasing doses of the agonist is required to obtain the same effect.

12. Which of the following is a pharmacodynamic property of a drug?

      (a)   Metabolism

      (b)   Absorption

      (c)   Receptor binding

      (d)   Protein binding

13. Which of the following would NOT delay the absorption of a drug from its site of injection?

      (a)   The addition of a vasodilator to the injection to increase blood flow through the site of injection

      (b)   Suspension of the active drug in oil (a 'depo' injection)

      (c)   Occlusion of the circulation in the area of the injection by use of a tourniquet

      (d)   Implantation of the drug in a solid pellet form under the skin

      (e)   Addition of a vasoconstrictor such as adrenaline to reduce blood flow through the site of injection

14. A drug that binds to a cell receptor and causes a response similar to an endogenous ligand is called an

      (a)   Agonist

      (b)   Antagonist

      (c)   Receptor blocker

      (d)   Partial agonist

15. Antihistamines work by

      (a)   Competitively inhibiting histamine at the receptor sites

      (b)   Chemically inactivating histamine

      (c)   Reversing the effects of histamine

      (d)   Blocking synthesis of histamine

16. Which of the following is an example of drugs with non-specific action?
    (a) Calcium channel blockers preventing the influx of calcium into vascular cell membranes
    (b) Emollients to moisturise the skin
    (c) Anti-histamine binding to histamine H1 receptors to relieve hay fever symptoms
    (d) Antibiotics inhibiting bacterial cell wall synthesis
17. Which of the following is NOT true about the site of action of a ligand?
    (a) It may act at the site of its secretion.
    (b) It may act at a site distant from its site of secretion.
    (c) It may act at a site on a single nerve cell across the synaptic space.
    (d) Only acts on enzymes responsible for excretion of drug metabolites in the kidney.
18. Which of the following is unlikely to be effective against bacteria?
    (a) Nystatin
    (b) Penicillin
    (c) Tetracycline
    (d) Ciprofloxacin
19. Drugs are often protein bound in the bloodstream, which of the following is the principal protein to which drugs are bound?
    (a) Albumen
    (b) Gamma globulin
    (c) Albumin
    (d) Fibrinogen
20. Which of the following may NOT reduce the duration of a drug's effect?
    (a) Extensive plasma protein binding of the drug
    (b) Increased renal excretion of the drug
    (c) Increased metabolism of the drug
    (d) Reduced plasma protein binding
21. Drugs with low lipid solubility may be transported across the cell membrane by combining
    (a) With a partial agonist
    (b) With a carrier molecule
    (c) With an agonist
    (d) With an antagonist
22. The main route of administration of a drug to provide a systematic effect is NOT
    (a) Topical
    (b) Oral
    (c) Parenteral
    (d) Transdermal
23. Which of the following is not necessary for the process of absorption?
    (a) Passive diffusion across a concentration gradient
    (b) Active transport of ions and water-soluble drugs
    (c) Lipid solubility so as to cross the cell membrane
    (d) Synthesis of hormones

24. An understanding of the principles of absorption helps the prescriber to decide on the most appropriate route of administration of a drug. Which of the following is NOT correct?
    (a) Topical application is appropriate for lipid soluble drugs where a local effect is desired.
    (b) Parenteral administration is appropriate in emergencies where the highest possible plasma levels are required immediately.
    (c) Poorly lipid soluble drugs, such as NSAIDs applied to the skin on an arthritic joint will reach therapeutic concentrations at the site of action within the joint.
    (d) Suppositories and enemas are used to deliver drugs directly to the site of action in and around the colon.
25. Drugs are metabolised principally in the
    (a) Stomach
    (b) Liver
    (c) Colon
    (d) Kidneys

Resources to support prescribers in keeping up to date with pharmacology

Non-medical prescribers need to ensure that they have access to appropriate training, support and CPD material in order to keep up to date with developments in pharmacology. Employing organisations have a duty to provide non-medical prescribers with access to these resources.

At the Nottingham University Lymn *et al.* (2008) have developed a range of reusable online learning objects, which are freely available according to creative commons conventions for educational use. These consist of a range of learning units on the basis principles of pharmacology and can be accessed at http://www.nottingham.ac.uk/nursing/sonet/rlos/bioproc/synapse/.

Perhaps the most valuable and accessible resource is the BNF, which is a joint publication of the British Medical Association (BMA) and the Royal Pharmaceutical Society of Great Britain (RPSGB). It is published biannually and aims to provide prescribers with thorough and up to date information on the legal and clinical use of medicines. It is an important reference for dosages, interactions and contraindications and guidelines on reporting adverse drug reactions (ADRs). The BNF consists of 15 chapters related to a particular system of the body and each chapter is further divided into sections to include clinical summaries of conditions and relevant drugs and preparations. The BNF also includes appendices on interactions, the older patient and pregnancy, breast feeding and renal impairment.

Table 7.2   Hierarchy of evidence.

Level of evidence	Example
(1)	Meta-analysis, systematic review of randomised controlled trial (RCT)
(2)	Case control and cohort studies; systematic reviews
(3)	Non-analytical studies, e.g. case reports, case series
(4)	Expert opinion

There is a lot of literature available, which can become overwhelming when trying to stay up to date with pharmacology. Original papers only need to be read occasionally when assessing a particular piece of evidence. Evidence-based practice and, in particular, formulating answerable questions is discussed in more detail in Chapter 3. As a basic rule for assessing the validity of evidence it is essential to remember the hierarchy of evidence as seen in Table 7.2.

It will come as no surprise to the prescriber that there are vast amounts of information sources in relation to medicines. The most accessible source is often other colleagues and there is evidence to suggest that most clinical research-based knowledge is disseminated by interpersonal contact. However, this should not be undervalued; sometimes it is necessary to refer to the literature for published research to inform prescribing practice further. This is not an easy task. There are thousands of journals published every year and books may go out of date quickly. Other sources are libraries and the Internet via the World Wide Web.

There are now a number of resources available, which provide readily appraised research, for example, *The Cochrane Database* of systematic reviews (Appendix 9). A systematic review is a review or summary of the literature in which evidence on a topic has been systematically identified, appraised and summarised according to pre-determined criteria. The reviewer includes not only the published but also, where available, unpublished literature.

The National Library for Health – This is currently a gateway for the following databases although they can also be accessed via National Health Service (NHS) Libraries (http://www.nlh.nhs.uk).

Cochrane Library – This was set up to provide systematic reviews of research on important areas of health care. It now covers most areas of health care. It is a very useful resource for prescribers because it discusses treatment options and is an invaluable source of information and would be recommended as your starting point.

Medline – This is the computerised version of Index Medicus. It contains a vast amount of information from thousands of biomedical journals.

British Nursing Index (BNI) – This is a British index of nursing articles, which is very useful. These are not always research based and contents are not quality assured.

CINAHL – This large database covers details of articles related to nursing, health education and the allied professions. The contents are not quality assured.

Best Evidence – This is an electronic version of the Evidence-Based Series of journals.

Searching filtered databases requires a number of skills, which can be taught by NHS librarians. Filtered databases are not the only source of evidence-based information that may inform the prescriber. The Internet provides a range of other resources that are potentially relevant. For example, the NHS website http://www.nelm.nhs.uk contains an extensive A–Z of links to prescribing related websites.

From 30 April 2009, The National Library for Health will be replaced by NHS Evidence. In the Darzi report, *High Quality Care for All* (published in June 2008), NICE was asked to establish NHS Evidence, which is expected to be a key component in the drive to improve the standard and quality of care across the NHS.

NHS Evidence will provide access to a comprehensive evidence base for everyone in health and social care who makes decisions about treatments or the use of resources.

The National Prescribing Centre (NPC) http://www.npc.co.uk now provides the most comprehensive gateway to pharmacological resources for prescribers and it is possible to sign up for updates, which can be delivered into an e-mail inbox on a daily basis. The National prescribing centre offers a number of resources which includes competency framework for prescribers, which helps to outline standards and criteria for pharmacological knowledge for prescribers.

The use of reputable resources that summarise evidence and make it accessible at the point of care is a very reliable method to practice evidence-based prescribing.

Examples include the following:

- *MeReC* (2007), http://www.npc.co.uk/merec.htm provides a range of high quality resources useful to a wide range of health-care professionals. They provide concise, evidence-based information about the clinical use of drugs and medicines.
- *The Drug and Therapeutics Bulletin* (2007) http://www.dtb.bmj.com is produced on a monthly basis by the consumer association, which provides an independent overview of drugs and treatments for prescribers.

Clinical guidelines summarise findings from important studies within a specific clinical area and make recommendations about how clinicians such as prescribers should behave (Greenhalgh 2006). These can be invaluable to support decision making within practice.

Examples include the following:

- NICE (2007) (National Institute of Clinical Excellence; http://www.nice.org.uk)
- SIGN (2007) (Scottish Intercollegiate Guidelines Network; http://www.sign.ac.uk)
- CKS (Clinical Knowledge Summaries; http://.www.cks.nhs.uk)
- Bandolier (2007) (http://www.library.nhs.uk)

Maintaining current awareness

It is essential that non-medical prescribers maintain current awareness of pharmacology in the areas in which they prescribe. Bibliographic databases allow you to save searches relating to your prescribing area of interest. These searches can be saved and periodically re-run, often automatically with the results sent to you by email. Alternatively, several journals or information resources provide an email alerting service and automatically email you on a regular basis with the list of the most recent tables of contents, or when articles in your area of interest are published. This can save an enormous amount of time, and is an easy way to keep up to date. More information can be sought from your local library.

The National Network for non-medical prescribers has an email alert service that prescribers can sign up to via the NPC's website (National Prescribing Centre (NPC) 2007; http://www.npc.o.uk). In addition, there are several courses that are run for non-medical prescribers by universities or in individual specialities that are useful for maintaining current awareness of pharmacology in ones area of practice.

The pharmaceutical industry can help prescribers maintain an awareness of new products. However, promotional literature and research papers need to be critically appraised to ensure that they are valid information resources. For example, a research paper published with the support of the pharmaceutical industry may be less valid than that published by an independent body. It is essential that the prescriber does not prescribe inappropriately because of pressure from patients, colleagues or the pharmaceutical industry.

Key sources of support and advice

Key sources of support and advice can usually be found locally from colleagues and the hospital pharmacy medical information department.

Pharmaceutical industry medical information departments are also useful sources of information on specific products.

Non-medical prescribers can keep up to date in pharmacology by reflecting on their own practice, for example, by using case studies to review the pharmacology of the drugs they are prescribing as part of their CPD. These could be shared with colleagues to encourage debate and peer review on prescribing practice between medical and non-medical prescribers. If prescribing errors occur, it is good practice to use a root cause analysis tool to learn for future prescribing practice.

It is essential that non-medical prescribers have a network for support, reflection, and learning. It is useful to establish multi-professional links with other practitioners that work in the same specialist area, for example, through participation in multidisciplinary meetings, non-medical prescribing study groups, or case presentations as outlined in Chapter 4. Tools that can be used to improve practice include prescribing data, audit and feedback.

The role of the supervisory relationship

Supervisors are key in supporting and advising non-medical prescribers. They can be medical prescribers or more senior non-medical prescribers practising in the same speciality. Supervisors have a role in ensuring that non-medical prescribers keep up to date with pharmacology, and practice evidence-based prescribing in line with local and national standards.

Current awareness of pharmacology can be maintained by reviewing cases in an individual's practice with a supervisor. For example, supervisors could sit in on non-medical prescribers' clinics. At the end of the clinic, practice can be reviewed with constructive discussions on how practice could be developed, changed or improved.

The supervisory relationship needs to be open, non-threatening, honest and constructive. This allows for two-way communication between the non-medical prescribers and their supervisor. Such a relationship is key to the CPD of the non-medical prescriber.

Conclusion

It is important to keep up to date and remain familiar with pharmacology as applied to the non-medical prescribers' area of prescribing practice in order to remain competent, safe and effective as a prescriber. Initial training serves as an introduction to the subject but it is important to retain knowledge of the basic principles of pharmacology and have access to a good range of evidence-based prescribing resources.

Key learning points

- It is essential that non-medical prescribers have current pharmacological knowledge relating to the products they prescribe.
- Key elements of pharmacology include pharmacokinetics, pharmacodynamics, pharmacogenetics, adverse drug reactions an d interactions.
- It is important for the non-medical prescriber and those who support their CPD to consider creative ways to retain and review this knowledge.
- It is the responsibility of the non-medical prescriber to access evidence-based prescribing resources to support the continued development of knowledge of pharmacology and employers to support this.
- It is also useful to identify other key sources of support especially in the workplace and in particular the expertise of pharmacist colleagues and other prescribers as mentors.
- Reflection on practice-based prescribing case histories is a useful tool for keeping up to date with pharmacology.

Key resources in Section Three

- Useful websites
- Answers to pharmacology self-test.

References

Bandolier (2007) [Online] Available at: http://www.library.nhs.uk [Accessed 14 December 2007].

Banning, M.. (2004) Nurse prescribing, nurse education and related research in the United Kingdom: a review of the literature. *Nurse Education Today* 24: 420–427.

BMJ Best Treatments (2007a) [Online] Available at: http://www.besttreatments.bmj.com/btuk/home.jsp [Accessed 14 December 2007].

BMJ Clinical Evidence (2007b) [Online] Available at: http://www.clinicalevidence.bmj.com/ceweb/index.jsp [Accessed 14 December 2007].

Courtenay, M. and Latter, S. (2003) Effectiveness of nurse prescribing: a review of the literature. *Journal of Clinical Nursing* 13: 26–32.

Drug and Therapeutics Bulletin (2007) [Online] Available at: http://www.dtb.bmj.com [Accessed 14 December 2007].

Greenhalgh, T. (2006) *How to Read a Paper: the Basics of Evidence-Based Medicine*, 3rd edition, London, BMJ Books.

Lymn, J., Bath-Hextall, F. and Wharrad, H. (2008) Pharmacology education for nurse prescribing students – a lesson in reusable learning objects. *BMC Nursing* 7: 2.

McGavock, H. (2001a) Getting a drug into the body: absorption. *Prescriber* 12(18). Available at: http://www.escriber.com/Prescriber/Features.asp? ID=297&GroupID=37&Action=View [Accessed 14 December 2007].

McGavock, H. (2001b) Getting a drug to its site of action: distribution. *Prescriber* 12(19). Available at: http://www.escriber.com/Prescriber/Features.asp? ID=304&GroupID=37&Action=View [Accessed 14 December 2007].

McGavock, H. (2001c) Phase 2 drug metabolism and methods of excretion. *Prescriber* 12(21). Available at: http://www.escriber.com/Prescriber/ Features.asp?ID=323&GroupID=37&Action=View [Accessed 14 December 2007].

McGavock, H. (2001d) Inactivating drugs – phase 1 drug metabolism. *Prescriber* 12(20). [Online] Available at: http://www.escriber.com/Prescriber/ Features.asp?ID=321&GroupID=37&Action=View [Accessed 14 December 2007].

McGavock, H. (2001e) Receptor function and intercellular signalling. *Prescriber* 12(22). Available at: http://www.escriber.com/Prescriber/Features.asp? ID=339&GroupID=37&Action=View [Accessed 14 December 2007].

McGavock, H. (2001f) The central role of receptors in drug action. *Prescriber* 12(23). Available at: http://www.escriber.com/Prescriber/Features.asp? ID=347&GroupID=37&Action=View [Accessed 14 December 2007].

McGavock, H. (2002a) The principal targets for drug action. *Prescriber* 13(3). Available at: http://www.escriber.com/Prescriber/Features.asp? ID=377&GroupID=37&Action=View [Accessed 14 December 2007].

McGavock, H. (2002b) Antibacterial action and bacterial resistance. *Prescriber* 13(6). Available at: http://www.escriber.com/Prescriber/Features.asp? Action=View&ID=401&GroupID=37&Page=1 [Accessed 14 December 2007].

McGavock, H. (2002c) How to prevent adverse drug interactions. *Prescriber* 13(8). Available at: http://www.escriber.com/Prescriber/Features.asp? ID=422&GroupID=37&Action=View [Accessed 14 December 2007].

McGavock, H. (2002d) How to predict and avoid adverse drug reactions. *Prescriber* 13(10). Available at: http://www.escriber.com/Prescriber/ Features.asp?ID=443&GroupID=37&Action=View [Accessed 14 December 2007].

McGavock, H. (2002e) The scientific basis of prescribing in the elderly. *Prescriber* 13(4). Available at: http://www.escriber.com/Prescriber/Features.asp? ID=384&GroupID=37&Action=View [Accessed 14 December 2007].

MeReC (2007) [Online] Available at: http://www.npc.co.uk/merec. htm [Accessed 14 December 2007].

National Institute of Clinical Excellence (2007) [Online] Available at: http://www.nice.org.uk [Accessed 14 December 2007].

NPC (2001) *Maintaining Competency in Prescribing – An Outline Framework to Help Nurse Prescribers*. Liverpool, The National Prescribing Centre.

NPC (2003a) *Maintaining Competency in Prescribing - An Outline Framework to Help Pharmacist Supplementary Prescribers*. Liverpool, National Prescribing Centre.

NPC (2003b) *Maintaining Competency in Prescribing – An Outline Framework to Help Nurse Supplementary Prescribers*. Liverpool, National Prescribing Centre.

NPC (2004) *Competency Framework for Prescribing Optometrists May*. Liverpool, National Prescribing Centre.

National Prescribing Centre (2007) *Non Medical Prescribing*. [Online] Available at: http://www.npc.co.uk/non_medical.htm [Accessed 14 December 2007].

Nursing and Midwifery Council (2004) *Outline Curriculum for the Preparation of Nurses, Midwives & Health Visitors to Prescribe from the Extended Nurse Prescribers' Formulary*. London, NMC.

Nursing and Midwifery Council (2006) *Standards of Proficiency for Nurse and Midwife Prescribers*. London, NMC.

Offredy, M., Kendall, S. and Goodman, C. (2007) The use of cognitive continuum theory and patient scenarios to explore nurse prescribers' pharmacological knowledge and decision-making. *International Journal of Nursing Studies* 45(2008): 855–868.

Scottish Intercollegiate Guidelines Network (SIGN) (2007) [Online] Available at: http://www.sign.ac.uk [Accessed 14 December 2007].

Sodha, M., McGlaughlin, M., Williams, G. and Dhillon, S. (2002) Nurses' confidence & pharmacological knowledge: a study. *British Journal of Community Nursing* 7(6): 309–315.

Thomson, A. (2004a) Back to basics: pharmacokinetics. *The Pharmaceutical Journal* 272: 769–771. Available at: http://www.pjonline.com/pdf/cpd/pj_20040619_pharmacokinetics01.pdf [Accessed 14 December 2007].

Thomson, A. (2004b) Variability in drug dosage requirements. *The Pharmaceutical Journal* 272: 806–808. Available at: http://www.pjonline.com/pdf/cpd/pj_20040626_pharmacokinetics02.pdf [Accessed 14 December 2007].

8 Organising CPD for Non-Medical Prescribers in a General Practice Setting

Mandy Fry

Introduction

Non-medical prescribing is a substantial growth area in primary care. The increasing utilisation of service developments such as nurse triage and nurse-led chronic disease management clinics and the move to place more specialist services within primary care has seen non-medical prescribing as the next logical step, not the least by politicians (DH 2005). This chapter aims to explore the context of the non-medical prescriber in a general practice setting, and helps the practitioner to utilise current resources for maintaining continuing professional development, as well as offering some practical advice that might continue to support further development.

The science and art of medicine in general practice

Primary care is probably the one area of practice where non-medical prescribing remains the most controversial as patients present with potentially complex, undifferentiated illness. In this setting, making prescribing decisions means much more than familiarity with a portion of the British National Formulary (BNF); it means being comfortable with dealing with the uncertainty of the real, messy world of general practice. In this context, perhaps more than anything else, continuing to develop as a prescriber means continuing to develop as a professional practitioner where skills in consulting, making diagnoses and holding uncertainty are as important as keeping up to date with the latest evidence base (Avery & Pringle 2005; Avery & James 2007). It means recognising that:

'medicine is an imperfect science, an enterprise of constantly changing knowledge, uncertain information, fallible individuals, and at
the same time lives on the line. There is science in what we do, yes,
but also habit, intuition, and sometimes plain old guessing. The gap
between what we know and what we aim for persists. And this gap
complicates everything we do.'

(Gawande 2002; p. 7)

The dichotomy between the science of aspects of medicine, such as
pharmacology, and the art of professional practice can be uncomfortable. It does not fit with the current preoccupation with skills acquisition
and competency-based assessments within educational practice. Yet,
failing to recognise its existence will result in continuing distrust of
non-medical prescribing by our medical colleagues, for their clinical
practice confirms its existence almost every day (Schön 1983). In con-
trast, recognising these issues will ensure that non-medical prescribers
remain valued and trusted members of the practice team, ensuring that
the whole team works together effectively to improve patient care.

It has to be remembered that non-medical prescribing within the
general practice setting encompasses a potential variety of roles to
include practice nurses, nurse practitioners, district nurses, health visitors and specialist nurse roles, especially mental health nurses dealing
with treatments for addictions. Although allied health professional
non-medical prescribers are smaller in numbers than nurse non-medical
prescribers, it can also include pharmacists, chiropodists, podiatrists
and physiotherapists who may be attached to or employed by general
practice.

The role of professional artistry and building community

The best time to start thinking about how to maintain continuing professional development as a non-medical prescriber is whilst undertaking
the initial training course. It is easy to get caught up in the heavy
workload and time pressures of the assessments but building links
with other local practitioners will be time well spent. They may well
have come across similar barriers to practice that non-medical practitioners in training might experience and be able to share insights into
how to approach them. Building a community of local practitioners,
not all of whom may be studying at the same institution, will also
help practitioners to start to integrate their new role as a non-medical
prescriber within their overall professional development at an early
stage. It will also help to make sense of how the knowledge base and

skills acquisition of the prescribing course fits with the more complex world of practice.

The experience of non-medical prescribers within the general practice setting where I work is that this was a huge missed opportunity. They started the course full of good intentions but were then easily distracted by its academic demands. However, they now recognise that had they followed through on their initial intentions, they may have saved themselves work in the longer term as they would now be reaping the benefits of others' experience. Instead, rather than taking learning opportunities from those around them, they repeatedly face the same issues rather than resolving recurrent problems.

Building community will also help to ensure that non-medical prescribers start to use new skills as soon as is practicable and thus by 'engaging in doing and reflecting on the doing' (Fish & Coles 1998; p. 37) facilitate their own development as 'an enlightened practitioner – a professional in charge of his or her own professional work, thoughtful about ends and means, able and willing to investigate both, and accountable for *and* able to give an account of his or her practice' (Fish & Coles 1998; p. 284). It is this transformation of formal knowledge, by practice, into personal knowledge (Eraut 1994) that will equip non-medical prescribers to become competent, effective practitioners. So having built community, the next step in continuing professional development as a non-medical prescriber in primary care is to both recognise and utilise any of the opportunities that present themselves and to start prescribing.

Starting to prescribe in practice may be more difficult than it initially sounds (Latter *et al.* 2005). There may be practical obstacles such as reconfiguring practice computer systems to recognise the new skills and qualifications of non-medical prescribers. Or there may be organisational issues to overcome, such as the continuing scepticism of medical practitioners towards the new role and the expectations of patients. So in order to enhance opportunities for professional development it may well be that the non-medical prescriber will first have to educate others. This might include presentations to a patient participation group or writing for the practice newsletter explaining how this new role has the potential to enhance the patient journey (Box 8.1). It might also include reassuring medical colleagues that the non-medical prescriber is aware of the complexities of practice, that competence is more than the accumulation of competencies. Getting receptionists on board in a general practice is also a key task as it is they who control access to appointments for non-medical prescribers who are running clinics.

It may be worth reflecting upon how they have been educated in the past when practitioners have developed skills in new areas, such as triage and family planning, for example, that have broadened pre-existing roles.

Box 8.1 Informing colleagues about new non-medical prescribing roles in general practice

- **Patients** – patient participation group, announcement in practice newsletter, information for practice notice board or website
- **Medical colleagues** – practice meetings, critical event analysis
- **Nursing or allied health professional colleagues** – professional forums, examples of where non-medical prescribing has worked well, writing reflective accounts for publication in professional journals
- **Administration staff** – explain boundaries of role, identify appropriate situations or organise clinics where it is relevant to use prescribing skills.

Making the most of existing educational opportunities

Having made the most of opportunities to prescribe, the next step might well be to take advantage of the educational activities that are already well developed within general practice in the United Kingdom. This is particularly true where practitioners are fortunate enough to be employed within or attached to training practices that are already accustomed to functioning as learning establishments alongside the provision of good clinical care.

The New General Medical Services Contract (nGMS) (DH 2004) introduced payments for results not only into direct clinical care but also into organisational and educational aspects of practice. Of particular relevance to continuing professional development as a non-medical prescriber is the requirement for all practice employed clinical staff to have an annual appraisal. This is designed to be a constructive opportunity to review performance objectives, progress and skills and to identify learning needs in a protected environment. It is to be hoped that these learning needs will include a review of practitioners' needs in relation to prescribing practice, as there will already have been significant investment in the development of non-medical prescribing by the practice. The annual appraisal is an opportunity for the non-medical prescriber to develop a well-thought-out personal development plan, which should dovetail with the practice development plan and which the practitioner could ensure continues to enhance their own development as a non-medical prescriber as well as contributing to their overall professional development.

The other area in which the Quality and Outcomes Framework of nGMS may be helpful is in the requirement for the practice to undertake regular significant event analysis. These are designed to be multidisciplinary in nature and may relate to both negative and positive examples of practice, the idea being to discuss events and cases and reflect upon areas for change. Medication errors are a common cause of negative events and clearly these are of direct clinical relevance to the non-medical prescriber. Indeed it may be this association between prescribing and adverse events that has led to some of the medical profession's concerns about the safety of non-medical prescribing (DTB 2006). However, looking at examples of excellence such as palliative care in the community can also help to highlight to the rest of the practice team how non-medical prescribing has enhanced the patient experience. It may also help to identify possible areas of practice into which non-medical prescribers could further develop their role, and thus feed into the development of personal development plans via the appraisal system or less formally.

There are often numerous publications relevant to prescribing that practice may receive, and non-medical prescribers should ensure that they are included in the circulation list. Examples might be guidelines from microbiologists about antibiotic prescribing in light of local patterns of resistance or updates from local reproductive and sexual heath services. There may also be publications to which the practice subscribes, such as the *Drugs & Therapeutics Bulletin*.

It is also imperative that non-medical prescribers remain aware of any prescribing incentive schemes that the practice has signed up to and perhaps attend review meetings with the local Primary Care Trust (PCT) pharmacist (Box 8.2). There is a perception amongst the medical profession that non-medical prescribers are less inclined to consider cost when prescribing (Horton 2002). Attending meetings to review prescribing practice with the PCT pharmacist, and undertaking an audit (via prescribing and cost trend analysis–PACT data) of one's own prescribing practice are potential ways in which our medical colleagues can be assured that non-medical prescribers are committed to cost-effective prescribing. Both approaches to developing awareness of the cost impact of prescribing would also help to identify those areas for which non-medical prescribers are most comfortable prescribing and perhaps highlight some clinical areas where there is room for development. However, whilst the practitioner in primary care might be faced with a broad array of conditions, the non-medial prescribers should remain aware that there is no compulsion to become competent to prescribe from all areas of the BNF (Avery & Pringle 2005; Avery & James 2007). In addition to this, an audit might also help identify those clinical areas on which non-medical prescribing practitioners intend to focus the further development of practice.

Box 8.2 Making the most of educational opportunities in the general practice setting

- Annual general appraisal and development of personal development plan
- Practising significant analysis events that relate to prescribing
- Sharing of good practice or exemplars of when non-medical prescribing has enhanced the patient journey
- Accessing relevant circulars, bulletins and publications, which relate to prescribing
- Liaising with PCT pharmacist in order to analyse personal PACT data.

Mentoring and critical friendship

If, like the majority of non-medical prescribers in primary care, you are from a nursing background then you are probably already well aware of the role of reflection and clinical supervision in continuing professional development. For a non-medical prescriber from any discipline, however, forming a mentoring, supervisory and/or critical friendship relationship is an extension of this, which can be of benefit to all those participating.

For those fortunate to be working in community settings with other non-medical prescribers, even if not directly in general practice, the formation of a critical friendship such as that described by Campbell *et al.* (2004) may well be a core component of continuing professional development. The idea is that such an individual would be 'a peer, a colleague and an equal' (Campbell *et al.* 2004; p. 110) with the capacity to both support and challenge. Such a relationship might well be uncomfortable on occasions but would enable the sharing of experiences in a constructive environment, thus enhancing the reflection on action that might be undertaken. The idea is that the key learning dynamic is one of both high challenge and high support, as otherwise 'most of us, unless we feel uncomfortable, shaken or forced to look at ourselves, are unlikely to change. It is far easier to accept our current conditions and adopt the least line of resistance' (Johns 2000; p. 60). It is certainly possible to reflect on practice in isolation but 'it is difficult to sustain because of the difficulty in surfacing and transcending what may be our own distorted self-understandings ... keeping our vision directed towards new possibilities for understanding and action' (Johns 2000; p. 52). This is despite the availability of various reflective templates such as the Gibbs' reflective cycle (Gibbs 1998) or Johns' model for structured reflection (Johns 2000). Developing a critical friendship enables practitioners to remain focused on a particular area of professional development, in this instance, the role as a non-medical prescriber.

Within the general practice setting in which I work, one of the practice nurses who has recently qualified as a non-medical prescriber has made links with one of our district nurses who is in a similar position. This has enabled them to support one another in their new role, to share the overcoming of potential obstacles to prescribing and to encourage one another to attend any regional continuing professional development events that are organised.

Similarly, developing a mentoring relationship can be of enormous value in emancipating knowledge and forcing non-medical prescribers to reflect on their decision making and helping them to use the real world of practice as the learning milieu in which they can test out new insights and new ways of working. However such a relationship demands a certain level of commitment from the individual as it is all about relying on an ability to take ownership of the desire and capability to change. It is worth taking some time to consider how individual practitioners might go about choosing a potential mentor or critical friend, and encouraging the practice community to support this as a learning opportunity.

There are several issues that practitioners might consider when choosing a potential mentor. The first might be to decide whether it is appropriate to opt for a mentor who is an individual directly responsible for their line management, for example, one of the general practitioner's (GP) partners. There are clear advantages in choosing such a person as they will be familiar with the context of the individual prescriber's practice so there may be opportunities for taking a shared approach to tackling certain situations and it may increase mutual respect and enhance the working relationship.

A model that works well in one practice is that practice nurses have the opportunity to bring back patients in whom they have encountered difficult prescribing decisions to a joint clinic with one of the GPs. This enables joint decision making and reflection on action with the advantage of two different clinicians' perspectives on the situation. Sometimes though, opting for line managers as mentors can be problematic as the mentors may take a more paternalistic approach, seeing their role as one of moulding the practitioners towards their way of thinking and being reluctant to consider other ways of doing things. This can result from conflict over a sense of control but it can also lead to the avoidance of sharing some experiences and thus diminish the potential for learning.

The suitability of the mentor

It may be that within a specific practice setting there appears to be little scope for having a mentor who is not involved in line management, even if that is not what the non-medical prescriber might desire, given free choice. Under these circumstances it might be worth considering more inventive solutions to the situation. For example, if you are a practice nurse you might choose to work in partnership with one of the attached staff, such as a district nurse, who shares the prescribing role, each taking on the role of critical friend. This may be complemented by a mentoring relationship with one of the GPs that may then become more akin to clinical supervision. It might also be worth considering whether there are any salaried GPs in the practice who might be keen to get more involved. One similar example is when practices have developed links with a neighbouring practice in order to develop mentoring relationships for practice staff, and in which one of the GPs acts as mentor to the other practice's non-medical prescriber and vice versa, using videoed consultations as one of the main springboards for reflection.

One of the other issues that might be considered is what training and experience the proposed mentor has of working as a mentor. A good initial first step would be to determine what the other individual perceives to be the meaning of the term mentor as there is considerable debate within the literature about the terminology. Within some organisations mentoring refers simply to more experienced individuals passing on their accumulated wisdom to others; however, it can be much more than that. One good definition of coaching and mentoring is 'learning relationships which help people to take charge of their own development, to release their potential and to achieve results which they value' (Connor & Pokora 2007; p. 6). In this way it facilitates insight, learning and change, using the present as a springboard to the future and enables the mentee to take a strategic approach to their professional development. It means that the potential mentor does not need to be an expert in the subject for which the non-medical prescriber is seeking mentorship, but it is more a partnership of equals where the mentor's expertise lies in the process of mentoring (Rogers 2001).

Models of mentorship

In establishing the credentials of a potential mentor, it may be worth exploring what approach they would take to the role and whether they would use an established framework or model. It is by no means essential that the mentor does use a model but it may help to ensure that the relationship is focussed on development rather than on the mentor providing solutions, which may or may not be appropriate but which are certainly less likely to be effective as the practitioner does not have ownership of the solutions. Rigidly sticking to a framework or model can be equally detrimental and flexibility remains an important aspect of any mentoring relationship. Two models which can be particularly effective in a health-care setting are the GROW (Goal,

Reality, Options/Opportunity, Will/What Next) model and Egan's Skilled Helper model.

The GROW (Box 8.3) model (Whitmore 2002) is about GROWing people, performance and purpose based on context, skills and sequence. The framework thus unfolds as the context of being aware of the need and responsibility for change and the mentor using the skills of effective questioning and active listening. This results in the GROW sequence – Goals; what do you want? Reality – what is happening now? Options – what could you do now? Will – what will you do? Thus, it is a straightforward model to follow but it does rely on an individual being able to articulate the goals that might be achieved and this can potentially be quite restrictive.

Box 8.3 The GROW model for coaching

- **G**oals – what do you want?
- **R**eality – what is happening now?
- **O**ptions – what could you do now?
- **W**ill – what will you do?

Another model, and the one that I favour, is Egan's Skilled Helper model (Box 8.4) (Egan 2002). Again the relationship between wanting change and acting is highlighted and it is a solution-focused framework. There are three stages: What's going on (the present)? What solutions make sense for me (the future)? How do I get what I need or want (linking the present and the future)? There are two main goals, the first being to help clients manage their problems more effectively and to develop unused resources and missed opportunities more effectively and the second is to help clients become more effective at helping themselves. The advantages of this model are that it encourages very broad-based visionary thinking that can help tap into previously unexplored opportunities and choices before focussing on practical, achievable goals. It can therefore be particularly helpful when issues have been identified that need to be addressed but the practitioner has been unable to tease out goals that they want to achieve.

Box 8.4 The Egan skilled helper model

- What is going on (the present)?
- What solutions make sense for me (the future)?
- How do I get what I need or want (linking the present and the future)?

An effective mentoring relationship can be an incredibly empowering model as it challenges the practitioner to take ownership of both the issues and all the potential solutions. The Egan model also provides a helpful framework that is relatively easy to comprehend that could be recommended to an individual who has agreed to be a mentor but has no prior experience of such a relationship.

If the practitioner chooses a novice mentor then it would be sensible to at least recommend that they read about their new role, such as Connor and Pokora (2007), if they are not prepared to undertake any formal training. Such an investment of time will be well rewarded in terms of the quality of the mentoring relationship that is achieved, and its subsequent benefit for continuing professional development.

Conclusion

General practice is a fertile training ground for continuing professional development as a non-medical prescriber. As with any area of practice, however, it will involve a degree of motivation from the individual. It is also worth exploring what other practitioners have tried and found helpful as many practices will be more than willing to try out ideas such as mentoring but may not have any prior experience of setting up such schemes. They will, however, have valuable experience as to how other developments in practice have been introduced to the wider practice team and the patient population. As always it is worth reflecting on what has worked well in the past and seeking to modify it appropriately rather than trying to continually reinvent the wheel. So, talking to one another and utilising prescribing skills in practice will be a cornerstone of continuing professional development.

Key learning points

- For non-medical prescribers, working in the general practice setting offers a unique set of challenges.
- The non-medical prescriber in general practice should identify and make use of existing educational opportunities.
- The non-medical prescriber should aim to build relationships throughout their period of study, will support their continuing professional development as a qualified prescriber.
- Raising the profile of non-medical prescribing within the practice team develops mutual trust as well as opportunities for development.
- The development of strong mentoring and clinical supervisory relationships is key to continuing professional development in the general practice setting.

Key resources in Section Three

- Prescribing points – two examples of communication of prescribing issues in a primary care setting.

References

Avery, A. J. and James, V. (2007) Developing nurse prescribing in the UK. *British Medical Journal* 335: 316.

Avery, A. J. and Pringle, M. (2005) Extended prescribing in the UK by nurses and pharmacists. *British Medical Journal* 331: 1154–1155.

Campbell, A., McNamara, O. and Gilroy, P. (2004) *Practitioner Research and Professional Development in Education.* London, Paul Chapman Publishing.

Connor, M. and Pokora, J. (2007) *Coaching and Mentoring at Work: Developing Effective Practice.* Maidenhead, Open University Press.

Department of Health (2004) *The New GMS Contract – Investing in General Practice.* London, The NHS Confederation and British Medical Association.

Department of Health (2005) *Improving Patients Access to Medicines: A Guide to Implementing Nurse & Pharmacist Independent Prescribing Within the NHS in England.* http://www.dh.gov.uk/en/Publicationsandstatistics/Publications/PublicationsPolicyAndGuidance/DH_4133743.

DTB (2006) Non-medical prescribing. *Drugs & Therapeutics Bulletin* 44: 33–37.

Egan, G. (2002) *The Skilled Helper,* 7th edition. Belmont, CA, Thomson Brooks/Cole.

Eraut, M. (1994) *Developing Professional Knowledge and Competence.* London, Falmer Press.

Fish, D. and Coles, C. (Eds) (1998) *Developing Professional Judgement in Health Care – Learning through the Critical Appreciation of Practice.* Oxford, Butterworth-Heinemann.

Gawande, A. (2002) *Complications: A Surgeon's Notes on an Imperfect Science.* London, Profile Books.

Gibbs, G. (1998) *Learning by Doing: A Guide to Teaching and Learning Methods.* Oxford, Oxford Brookes University, Further Education Unit.

Horton, R. (2002) Nurse prescribing in the UK: right but also wrong. *The Lancet* 359: 1875–1876.

Johns, C. (2000) *Becoming a Reflective Practitioner – A Reflective and Holistic Approach to Clinical Nursing, Practice Development and Clinical Supervision.* Oxford, Blackwell Publishing.

Latter, S., Maben, J., Myall, M., Courtenay, M., Young, A. and Dunn, N. (2005) *An Evaluation of Extended Formulary Independent Nurse Prescribing.* Southampton, University of Southampton, Department of Health.

Rogers, J. (2001) *Adults Learning.* Buckingham, Open University Press.

Schön, D. A. (1983) *The Reflective Practitioner – How Professionals Think in Action.* Hampshire, Ashgate Publishing Ltd.

Whitmore, J. (2002) *Coaching for Performance; GROWing People, Performance and Purpose,* 3rd edition. London, Nicholas Brealey.

9 Organising and Running a Journal Club for Non-Medical Prescribers

Dan Lasserson

Introduction

How can we improve our practice? How can we get answers to questions that arise when we see patients? How can we get research into practice? A journal club can help in finding the answers to these questions. Organising and running a journal club is not just about setting up a regular meeting – it is about a whole way of practice that gives you the freedom to ask questions and the power to help answer them.

A journal club can help in the delivery of evidence-based practice. There are increasing expectations that health-care interventions should be based upon evidence – in other words, there should be a reason why we believe that one form of treatment may be better than another. For the non-medical prescriber, the most common sort of evidence that will answer questions about prescribing will be in the form of a randomised controlled trial. The journal club process will help in finding the right sort of evidence and provide a framework for appraising research. How that research is then used to change practice is not straightforward but we need to be as concerned with strategies to change health care as we are with tracking down and discussing evidence (Glasziou & Haynes 2005).

Why run a journal club and what makes them effective?

All health-care professionals will at some stage come across a clinical problem where previous training or guidelines do not provide answers.

There may be no obvious source of expertise to ask for solutions. However, answers to problems may lie in the enormous amount of international research that is published week by week.

The 'old school' journal club has been seen as a rather stuffy academic exercise with little bearing on day-to-day decision making needed for effective patient care (Hatala *et al.* 2006). A journal club should have patient care as its focus rather than merely practising the skills of critically appraising papers. This is reflected in the definition of evidence-based practice by one of its pioneers, David Sackett, who stresses the integration of the individual clinician's experience with the best available evidence and incorporating the values and concerns of the patient (Sackett *et al.* 1996).

Journal clubs are not effective if they are stand-alone entities. As such, they do not facilitate the development of evidence-based practice and do little to change clinician's clinical behaviours (Coomarasamy & Khan 2004). Teaching how to appraise research in specific clinical contexts has had greater success in the development of evidence-based practice.

Providing access to information at the right time has a crucial bearing on use of evidence in practice. 'Point of care' access to research, that is, quick and easy availability of searching tools has improved evidence use. McGinn *et al.* (2002) found that 75% of clinicians, who were trained in using a system to allow them immediate access to research evidence at the bedside, would use evidence in the future. Straus *et al.* (2005) demonstrated an increase in the use of proven therapies in clinical practice from 49% to 62% of consecutive patients in a district hospital by improving access to electronic searches as well as providing training in evidence-based medicine.

Is integrating evidence-based practice, including journal clubs, into clinical contexts enough to support long-term improvements in use of evidence among health-care workers? Although demand for teaching of evidence-based practice is high (Leipzig *et al.* 2003), initial teaching does not seem to be enough for the maintained use of evidence in practice. Yew and Reid (2008) assessed doctors' practice 5 years after completing evidence-based medicine modules. Disappointingly there was little use of evidence, even amongst those who agreed strongly with the use of evidence and could demonstrate sound knowledge of evidence-based practice. The main barriers to using evidence were time and pressures of clinical practice.

Thus, running a journal club can only succeed in delivering evidence-based practice if the research discussed is aimed at solving a clinical problem. Those taking part in the journal club need to have easy access to research databases as well as training in how to use them. Protected time is essential to facilitate the process of translating research into practice, and this has been found to be a barrier to implementing evidence among nurses in the United States (Fink *et al.* 2005). Without methods of logging clinical problems that drive the searching of research literature, opportunities for real improvement in clinical practice will be lost. As yet, there is no model of delivering evidence-based practice, which has a proven track record of sustainable behavioural change amongst health-care workers. A well run journal club, however, is a good place to start.

How does this relate to non-medical prescribers?

In Latter *et al.*'s qualitative study of nurse-prescribers educational needs, newly qualified practitioners were asked about what they thought was central to education and practice in their new role (Latter *et al.* 2007). Although 55% reported that they knew where to get 'information' from, no specific questions were asked about how to find or use evidence in relation to clinical problems and no dominant themes emerged about evidence-based practice or running journal clubs.

Banning (2005) concludes that evidence-based practice is central to nurse prescribing and the training of nurse prescribers should include appraising evidence from randomised controlled trials. Although nurse prescribers were aware of the principles of research in this qualitative study they did not personally read research papers and were not familiar with the mechanics of evidence-based practice.

Melnyck *et al.* (2008) suggested that there is a knowledge gap in teaching strategies in evidence-based practice, from a qualitative analysis of interviews with nurse practitioner educators. The authors conclude that integrated evidence-based practice was required in speciality courses, to set the model for the future of specialist nurse care.

However, Holmes *et al.* (2006) pits the evidence of evidence-based practice against the complex care that nurses deliver. The criticism here is that the evidence hierarchy which places randomised controlled trials and meta-analyses above individual experience and studies of personal responses may not help decision making about complex areas of nursing practice.

The hierarchy that evidence-based practice applies to nursing is also challenged by Mantzoukas (2008), in a comparison with reflective nursing practice. Their main argument against the use of evidence-based practice is that the expert practitioner is removed from being able to define what best practice is in his or her nursing speciality – the ownership of the speciality is given over to 'researchers, academics and educationalists' who, they say, are not involved with daily practice.

However, evidence-based practice if done well is embedded in the clinician's experience and the patient's concerns. Thinking through the results of a trial and whether it applies to your patient is a key feature of linking research with practice. If practitioners are supported in using research to help answer questions about their practice such as in a regular journal club then arguably they are defining what counts as 'best practice' and not the people who carried out the research.

Organising a journal club

There is no 'one size fits all' approach in organising a journal club. The best method of organisation is by consensus. Initially, there should be an open invitation to take part amongst anyone working in the health-care team in the local environment, for example, community health centre. A discussion about the benefits of a journal club is important as people will need to give time not just for the discussion itself but also time reading the journal article and developing the skills of critical appraisal. The above discussion of how journal clubs and evidence-based practice are linked as well as counter-arguments to criticisms of the processes involved may help you in conversations with colleagues.

As discussed in Doust *et al.* (2008), the local workflow pattern and established meeting times may suggest the optimal time for the journal club to meet. Some general practitioner (GP) practices meet before the start of surgery for a 'working breakfast' while others fit it into a rota of different weekly lunchtime meetings. With agreement on the benefits of a journal club, time can be found for regular meetings.

As with any regular meeting, things run more smoothly if a nominated person is responsible for establishing the schedule of meetings. A degree of administrative support is helpful for the dissemination of articles for the group before the club meets, as well as in recording the outcomes of the discussion for the journal club log.

Running a journal club

The challenges in the running of a journal club are in maintaining the momentum and enthusiasm of the group. Hopefully as the experience of a journal club progresses, practitioners will see the benefit in terms of a fresh look at their own practice as well as the personal enrichment that learning new skills brings.

A key part of building up the journal club is facilitating an environment where anyone feels they can contribute not only to the discussion about research and changing clinical practice but also in terms of bringing their own questions and research as a focus for a club meeting. This is where a journal club acts as a powerful tool for multidisciplinary learning.

What skills do people need to take part?

Anyone who is interested in health care can take part in a journal club. The essential requirement is an inquiring mind. Successful journal clubs have participants who are comfortable asking 'why' questions about health-care interventions, e.g., 'why use this drug over that one?' or 'why use any drug at all – don't other things work?'.

The skills needed for a successful journal club are not complicated and can be developed with practice. A number of courses are run by UK universities and are pitched at absolute beginners from all backgrounds, clinical and non-clinical and can be very helpful in meeting learning needs in evidence-based practice.

Finding research to discuss in a journal club

A piece of research should help you answer a question about your practice, perhaps a patient you have seen or from general reflection about particular conditions and their treatments. All of us have thoughts about this but how often do we make an effort to write questions somewhere?

Capturing questions is the first step in finding the right piece of research for discussion. This could be in a log either held by an individual practitioner or perhaps held by the practice where different health-care team members can jot down ideas.

The form of the question about your practice will help in searching for journal papers. The key terms used to search research databases can be generated from a clinical scenario. The Centre for Evidence-Based Medicine at Oxford University uses a format based on Richardson *et al.* (1995) that easily translates clinical questions into a structure that makes searching for the right article simpler. It is termed *PICO* and consists of 'patients', 'intervention', 'comparison or comparator' and 'outcome' (Box 9.1). A worked example will illustrate this.

Box 9.1 PICO

> - **P**atients
> - **I**ntervention
> - **C**omparison or **c**omparator
> - **O**utcome.

Let us say that you saw a patient with type 2 diabetes and she wanted to know what you thought about recent newspaper reports about the safety of one of the drugs she was taking. She had become very concerned that there may be an increased risk of heart disease from drug 'X' and, as a result, she wanted to stop taking it. She is very aware that the control of her diabetes may not be as good without this drug and wants to know your opinion about whether or not to stay on drug 'X'.

The question that we need to answer here is 'what is the evidence that drug X increases heart disease in patients with type 2 diabetes?' (Box 9.2)

Box 9.2 PICO in detail

---

1. Patients (P)
What are the defining characteristics of the patient or group of patients? For example, many trials use patients that are as young and fit as possible (except for the condition of interest in the trial). As such the patient in front of you might not be representative of those in a particular trial. This may mean that conclusions that you draw from the results of the paper may not apply to the patient and therefore you cannot generalise the results. Of course, some characteristics are less important than others in determining generalisability of results. As a general rule, it is important to find research where participants closely match the kind of patients that you see.

2. Intervention (I)
The intervention is the active treatment, e.g. a novel drug that is being compared against either a placebo (a drug indistinguishable from the active drug but with no effects on the body) or some standard treatment, e.g. an older and well-established drug. In this example, drug X is the intervention, but you might be interested in different doses of X, particularly as harmful events might be related to the amount of drug taken.

3. Comparator (C)
Our question here is about the safety of drug X, but we would also be interested to know if being on it is less safe than the current alternative therapies in diabetes. As such it might be helpful if it was compared with other forms of treatment.

4. Outcome (O)
The key outcome we are interested in is the occurrence of heart disease. However, this includes a range of problems from heart failure to heart attack and is not very specific as a term to use in searching databases. A medical subject heading (MESH) term can be used here as a shorthand to include any heart problem in the search. Most drug trials, though, usually include any serious adverse event so that key trials are not likely to be missed.

Although the PICO mnemonic for search terms for trials does not include a 'T' for time, it is usually very important for thinking about how research relates to practice in drug trials. Patients with chronic diseases typically take medications for months or years, yet drug trials do not often provide results for these time frames.

Using PICO terms in an electronic search will yield a number of results in a MEDLINE or other database search and further specification may be needed, e.g. to limit the search to randomised controlled trials. These searching strategies can be honed with practice and help from your local health-care librarian or colleagues, as well as attending evidence-based practice courses. A number of workbooks and online resources further illustrate searching techniques (see Key Resources in Section Three, Appendix 9:1).

Presenting and discussing research at a journal club

It is often helpful to have a leader for each meeting to chair discussions. Doust *et al.* (2008) suggests that the person bringing a paper to the journal club presents the scenario that led them to ask a question not answered by their own knowledge base. This roots the paper in clinical practice and anchors later discussion to how practice could be changed, if at all. A good facilitator will also try to keep the discussion around the paper, rather than veering off on a tangent, as well as allowing all those who want to participate room to be heard.

Although it may seem sensible to distribute the paper under discussion before the club meets, Phillips and Glasziou (2004) found that most people did not read it and forgot to bring their copy to the meeting. Nevertheless they found that the journal club could still function with reading papers in the meeting as the majority of attendees were not made to feel left out.

The Centre for Evidence-Based Medicine at Oxford provides a useful structure for thinking about the quality of research trials (http://www.cebm.net/critical_appraisal.asp) as well as sheets to download, which can become the centrepiece for a journal club and filled out with key components of a trial as the discussion progresses. This will ultimately inform whether the trial that you found can help in answering your clinical question.

In order to believe the results of a trial we need to be confident that the researchers have done all they can to reduce bias – in other words, we need to be convinced that the results they found were only due to the intervention and not caused by some other factor. A higher quality trial will have done more to minimise the chance of bias.

The critical appraisal process looks at sources of bias. In the journal club discussion the important areas to cover are described in Box 9.3.

Box 9.3 Topics for discussion at a journal club

---

1. Randomisation
   Did participants in the trial have an equal chance of being given the intervention or the comparator? Was this done by a computer? Were the patients in the different groups similar?

2. **Allocation concealment**
   Did the patients and the researcher know which medicine they were given?
3. **Maintenance**
   Were participants treated equally apart from the different medications?
   Were all participants followed up until the end of the trial?
4. **Outcome measures**
   Was there something that could be measured reliably, e.g. change in laboratory values?

More information about the appraisal process can be found in various sources on line (e.g. http://www.cebm.net, http://www.jr2.ox.ac.uk/Bandolier/Extraforbando/Bias.pdf) and thinking about sources of bias gives structure to journal club discussions as well as prompts to ensure that the key areas that could influence translation of research into practice are covered.

The results section of a paper will also guide you as to whether it is worth changing practice to the drug or methods used in the research. The amount of benefit can be estimated from simple statistics, such as the 'number needed to treat' (NNT), which gives the number of patients that would need to be given a drug in order to prevent or cause a particular outcome of interest. These calculations can be seen 'in action' in every issue of the EBM journal (http://ebm.bmjjournals.com/collections), where evidence from trials in primary care or internal medicine is discussed and potential impacts presented in this way.

A log of journal club questions, research papers and discussion outcomes should be kept. This will form a record of the range of material considered as well as providing the opportunity for reflection about how your practice may have changed over time incorporating the outcomes of journal club discussions. Importantly, a log also provides part of a portfolio of evidence for professional appraisal.

Conclusion

Perhaps, the most important part of the journal club process is working out how to incorporate evidence into practice. As Kearley (2007) discusses, the formulation of an action plan starts in the journal club discussion but changes over time because changing practice is a complex intervention. Barriers to change exist but that should not dampen the fire of the evidence-based journal club.

Key learning points

- The journal club process will help in finding the right sort of evidence and provide a framework for appraising research.
- Teaching how to appraise research in specific clinical contexts has had greater success in the development of evidence-based practice.
- Running a journal club can only succeed in delivering evidence-based practice if the research discussed is aimed at solving a clinical problem.
- Those taking part in the journal club need to have easy access to research databases as well as training in how to use them.
- Evidence-based practice if done well is embedded in the clinician's experience and the patient's concerns. Thinking through the results of a trial and whether it applies to your patient is a key feature of linking research with practice.
- A key part of building up the journal club is facilitating an environment where anyone feels they can contribute.
- The form of the question about your practice will help in searching for journal papers. The key terms used to search research databases can be generated from a clinical scenario.
- The acronym 'PICO' can be used to integrate a question about your practice with database searching.
- It is often helpful to have a leader for each journal club meeting to chair discussions.
- A number of online resources provide critical appraisal frameworks, which can be downloaded and used in journal club meetings.
- A log of journal club questions, research papers and discussion outcomes should be kept.
- The most important part of the journal club process is working out how to incorporate evidence into practice.

Key resources in Section Three

- Developing a search strategy based on 'PICO'.

References

Banning, M. (2005) Conceptions of evidence, evidence-based medicine, evidence-based practice and their use in nursing: independent nurse prescribers' views. *Journal of Clinical Nursing* 14(4): 411–417.

Coomarasamy, A. and Khan, K. S. (2004) What is the evidence that postgraduate teaching in evidence based medicine changes anything? A systematic review. *British Medical Journal* 329: 1017–1021.

Doust, R., Del Mar, C., Montgomery, B. *et al.* (2008) EBM journal clubs in general practice. *Australian Family Physician* 37: 54–56.

Fink, R., Thompson, C. and Bonnes, D. (2005) Overcoming barriers and promoting the use of research in practice. *The Journal of Nursing Administration* 35(3): 121–129.

Glasziou, P. and Haynes, B. (2005) The paths from research to improved health outcomes. *ACP Journal Club* 142: A8–10.

Hatala, R., Keitz, S., Wilson, M. and Guyatt, G. (2006) Beyond journal clubs. Moving toward an integrated evidence-Based medicine curriculum. *Journal of General Internal Medicine* 21: 538–541.

Holmes, D., Perron, A. and O'Byrne, P. (2006) Evidence, virulence, and the disappearance of nursing knowledge: a critique of the evidence-based dogma. *Worldviews Evidence-Based Nursing* 3(3): 95–102.

Kearley, K. (2007) The 6 steps of evidence-based medicine: action plans and changing clinical practice through journal clubs. *Evidence Based Medicine* 12: 98–100.

Latter, S., Maben, J., Myall, M. and Young, A. (2007) Evaluating nurse prescribers' education and continuing professional development for independent prescribing practice: Findings from a national survey in England. *Nurse Education Today* 27: 685–696.

Leipzig, R. M., Wallace, E. Z., Smith, L. G., Sullivant, J., Dunn, K. and McGinn, T. (2003) Teaching evidence-based medicine: a regional dissemination model. *Teaching and Learning in Medicine* 15(3): 204–209.

Mantzoukas, S. (2008) A review of evidence-based practice, nursing research and reflection: levelling the hierarchy. *Journal of Clinical Nursing* 17: 214–223.

McGinn, T., Seltz, M. and Korenstein, D. (2002) A method for real-time, evidence based general medical attending rounds. *Academic Medicine* 77: 1150–1152.

Melnyk, B. M., Fineout-Overholt, E., Feinstein, N. F., Sadler, L. S. and Green-Hernandez, C. (2008) Nurse practitioner educators' perceived knowledge, beliefs, and teaching strategies regarding evidence-based practice: implications for accelerating the integration of evidence-based practice into graduate programs. *Journal of Professional Nursing* 24(1): 7–13.

Phillips, R. and Glasziou, P. (2004) What makes evidence-based journal clubs succeed? *Evidence Based Medicine* 9: 36–37.

Richardson, W. S., Wilson, M. C., Nishikawa, J. and Hayward, R. S. (1995) The well-built clinical question: a key to evidence-based decisions. *ACP Journal Club* 123: A12–A13.

Sackett, D., Rosenberg, W. M. C., Muir Gray, J. A., Haynes, R. B. and Richardson, W. S. (1996) Evidence based medicine: what it is and what it isn't. *British Medical Journal* 312: 71–72.

Straus, S. E., Ball, C., Balcombe, N., Sheldon, J. and McAlister, F. A. (2005) Teaching evidence-based medicine skills can change practice in a community hospital. *Journal of General Internal Medicine* 20(4): 340–343.

Yew, K. S. and Reid, A. (2008) Teaching evidence-based medicine skills: an exploratory study of residency graduates' practice habits. *Family Medicine* 40(1): 24–31.

Further reading

Glasziou, P., Mar, C. D. and Salisbury, J. (2003) *Evidence Based Medicine Workbook – Finding and Applying the Best Research Evidence to Improve Patient Care*. Oxford, Wiley Blackwell.

Heneghan, C. and Badenoch, C. (2006) *Evidence-Based Medicine Toolkit*. Wiley Blackwell.

Useful websites

http://www.cochrane.org/index.htm
http://www.jr2.ox.ac.uk/Bandolier
http://www.york.ac.uk/healthsciences/centres/evidence/cebn.htm
http://www.cebm.net

Section Three

Key Resources and Practice Examples for Non-Medical Prescribers

Introduction

Our aim in this section has been to accumulate resources that are excellent examples of material that is currently in use, to illustrate the amount of activity that is being undertaken to provide continuing professional development for non-medical prescribers. These resources range from a list of useful and authoritative websites that relate to each of the chapters, to evaluation tools, examples of update circulars produced by primary care and acute Trusts and illustrated examples of teaching and learning sessions. We are very grateful to the authors of the resources in this section, whose contribution is acknowledged, for the permission to re-print their work.

Each appendix relates to a numbered chapter, and the resources contained within the appendix can be used either in relation to the chapter to illustrate examples of good practice, or can be used as a stand-alone example that can be transferred to the reader's context, as a non-medical prescriber, manager or organisational lead.

APPENDIX 1

Key Resources for Keeping Up to Date with Legal and Professional Frameworks for Non-Medical Prescribing

This appendix relates to Chapter 1 and includes a list of useful websites, where the reader is able to access key resources that relate to legal and professional frameworks. An example job description and person specification is included to enable the reader to view a 'living' example of a job description that includes non-medical prescribing as a key requirement of the role. This is not prescriptive, but offers an example of how non-medical prescribing can be incorporated clearly into a job description.

A final part to this appendix offers the correct answers to the 'test your knowledge' quiz in Chapter 1.

1:1   Useful websites

Health Professions Council (HPC)
  http://www.hpc-uk.org/index.asp
Medicines and Healthcare Regulatory Agency (MHRA)
  http://www.mhra.gov.uk/index.htm
NHS Education Scotland (NES) CPD tool for non-medical prescribing
  http://www.nes.scot.nhs.uk
The National Prescribing Centre (NPC) current awareness daily bulletins
  http://www.npc.co.uk/ecab/ecab.htm
The National Prescribing Centre, Competency Frameworks
  http://www.npc.co.uk/prescribers/competency_frameworks.htm

The National Prescribing Centre Guide for Managers
  http://www.npc.co.uk/policy/publications/publications.htm?
  type=all
The Nursing and Midwifery Council (NMC)
  http://www.nmc-uk.org/
The Royal College of Ophthalmologists. Independent Prescribing for
  Optometrists
  http://www.rcophth.ac.uk/standards/independent-prescribing
The Royal Pharmaceutical Society of Great Britain (RPGSB) CPD Template
  plate
  http://www.uptodate.org.uk/home/PlanRecord.shtml

1:2   Example job description that includes non-medical prescribing as a key element of the role

Job description of consultant nurse/midwife

Job Title:	Consultant nurse/midwife
Grade:	Consultant nurse/midwife
Accountable to:	Directorate manager/Director of midwifery
Responsible to:	Director of nursing and clinical leadership
Key relationships:	Divisional and directorate clinical directors, consultant medical staff, matrons, deputy and associate directors of nursing and clinical leadership

Job summary

Responsibilities of a consultant nurse/midwife include the following:

- To provide inspirational leadership for nurse-/midwifery-led care within the Trust
- To be an expert nurse/midwife, providing leadership to nurses/ midwives that promotes and improves quality of care for clients and their families
- To actively participate in advancing nursing/midwifery practice at a strategic level and through expertise in nursing/midwifery practice
- To facilitate the provision of interdisciplinary care for patients using the post holder's area of professional expertise in the NHS Trust.

Post holders will contribute to the professional development of their field at local, national and international levels. They will provide nursing/midwifery expertise for patients, families and caregivers.

The post holder will lead the curriculum development activity, developing and providing educational activities using advanced and wide-ranging professional expertise to support the development of effective, evidence-based multidisciplinary clinical practice.

The post holder will be responsible for providing high-level expert advanced practice through leadership, consultation, clinical advice, teaching, research and mentorship/support for staff. **They will advise on diagnosis and prognosis and will prescribe treatment for patients/clients with complex clinical conditions, across specialities and divisions.** They will lead nursing/midwifery research, audit and evaluation. They will work collaboratively with the local universities, the NHS Trust, ambulance services and the PCT to ensure the successful development and application of knowledge, research and skills across the patient/client pathway to achieve high-quality clinical outcomes.

The post holder will ensure a dynamic response to the changing needs in their field of professional expertise, taking a professional lead in the establishment of an evidence-based approach to practice, and fostering a culture that contributes to the clinical governance agenda. The specific functions of the role will require the post holder to liaise with multi-professional colleagues across the Trust and through external organisations.

This post is based in clinical practice and involves working directly with patients, clients or communities for at least 50% of the time. The post integrates four core functions outlined below. These should not be viewed as discrete, but as closely inter-related elements of a coherent whole.

Core functions

Expert practice function

- Provide expert care for patients/clients and their caregivers using the post holder's expertise.
- Manage, direct and/or coordinate the care of patients, involving multi-professional colleagues across the Trust departments and sites.
- Advise and consult with patients/clients and their carers, to facilitate diagnosis and early recognition of symptoms and to promote timely interventions in treatment and self-care.
- Exercise professional autonomy and make critical judgments of the highest order in their field of expertise.
- Make decisions where precedents do not exist where appropriate without recourse to others, advising and supporting colleagues in the management of patients where standard protocols do not apply.
- Develop and implement protocols and guidelines for patient/client care and management across the patient journey from primary through secondary and tertiary care, and follow-up as necessary.

- Draw on advanced knowledge and exercise professional skills, working across traditional professional and service boundaries, in order to expedite assessment and decision making in relation to the management of patients/clients.
- Develop sustainable services for patients/clients and their carers.
- Make and receive referrals.
- Exercise independent prescribing rights.
- Use advanced skills to communicate specialist and complex clinical information to patients/clients, their carers, family and staff.
- Maintain accurate and legible patient/client records appropriate to the specialist area and expert level of practice.
- Lead the development of non-medical prescribing protocols in relation to the management of patients/clients.

Professional leadership and consultancy function

- Operate in a senior strategic and practice-based position, providing a significant professional leadership function.
- Provide expert clinical leadership and vision to strategic developments in the Trust that relate to local, national and international trends and demands.
- Formulate long-term plans that may involve uncertainty, and which may impact across the organisation and beyond.
- Respond to ad hoc requests for advice, support and guidance from individuals or teams.
- Exercise professional and clinical leadership skills to promote best practice.
- Support, supervise, mentor and inspire colleagues to improve quality and professional practice.
- Develop policy, standards, protocols, systems and competence for managing evidence-based care utilising leadership and change management skills of the highest order, through local, national, and international inter-professional liaison.
- Take a leading role in clinical governance, providing expert input to secure quality improvement.
- Influence other disciplines and the wider organisation across organisational boundaries, to deliver better services and seamless care.
- Provide expert advice across all disciplines, acting as a resource to others and providing facilitative support within the organisation and through liaison with internal and external agencies.
- Influence the national and international policy agenda by membership of working parties, networking with professional colleagues and other agencies.
- Act as an advocate for service users at local, regional and national levels.

Education, training and development function

- Utilise professional knowledge and expertise in education, training and development across professions.
- Identify and respond to learning needs at individual, team and organisational levels, particularly focusing on experienced colleagues, to develop advanced knowledge and skills.
- Play a key role to integrate theory and practice through formal, informal methods including clinical educational opportunities.
- Establish and maintain formal university partnerships to support and advance the aims of the profession and provide the academic and research support needed.
- Play a key role in leadership and professional development through modelling, mentorship and clinical supervision.
- Support colleagues undertaking higher level and postgraduate studies by acting as a mentor and personal professional academic supervisor and through nurturing and developing advanced scholarly activity.

Practice and service development, research and evaluation function

- Develop professional practice locally and nationally through professional associations and other forums.
- Constructively challenge practice that is creating barriers to agreed standards of care.
- Promote evidence-based practice.
- Lead in setting, monitoring and auditing of standards, including those set locally and nationally.
- Identify and promote measures to secure and evaluate quality improvement.
- Innovate when necessary to deal with ambiguous, unique, or novel problems, and thereby create precedents, generate, monitor and evaluate new practice protocols.
- Benchmark local services against the highest national and international standards in the specialty.
- Initiate and evaluate the implementation of regional and national policy relevant to the area of practice.
- Maintain a track record of scholarship and the appraisal and application of research in practice, leading and developing clinical research relevant to the role and the context in which care is provided.
- Lead and develop clinical, practice or health service research relevant to the role and the context in which care is provided.

- Develop and contribute to programmes of clinical, practice or health services research.
- Lead nursing/midwifery in reviewing national guidance as it relates to care in the post holder's area of expertise, and establish programmes for auditing, implementing and evaluating change.

This job description will be reviewed with the post holder in accordance with the NHS Trusts developments in Clinical Services Specialities.

Person specification for consultant nurse/midwife post

Specification	Essential	Desirable
1. Education/ Training	• Current registration with the Nursing and Midwifery Council (NMC) on a part of the register relevant to the field • Evidence of significant post-registration development in the field • Possession of a National Board-approved qualification recordable with the NMC • Possession of a recordable teaching qualification • PhD • Working at doctoral level, or equivalent • **Registered independent/supplementary non-medical prescriber**	
2. Relevant experience	• A portfolio of career-long learning, experience and formal education, usually up to or beyond masters degree level • Research experience • A record of scholarship and publication • Substantial post-registration experience with relevant recent senior experience in the field • Evidence of effective leadership in a senior clinical position • A track record of practice development and scholarship sufficient to have inspired recognition as an expert and innovator in the field • Proven track record in operational management/team building skills	

3. Relevant Special skills/aptitudes	• The individual should have the following personal attributes necessary to function effectively in senior and influential posts:
	  ○ Confidence
	  ○ Good interpersonal skills
	  ○ Team player
	  ○ Tactful and diplomatic
	  ○ Integrity
	  ○ Articulate	

Specification	Essential	Desirable
	• Evidence of collaboration and cooperation with others in a team • Evidence of the ability to hold a clear strategic vision and develop implementation plans • Ability to work and communicate effectively within a multi-disciplinary forum and with other professionals • Ability to educate and inspire multi-professional audiences • Good organisational skills – in terms of coordinating work, educating patients, assuring the quality of care delivery and liaising with other professionals	
4. Special requirement	• Excellent leadership skills • Handles criticisms maturely • Commitment to high quality patient focused service • Ability to organise work around competing demands for time • Proactive organisational skills • Flexible working pattern	

1:3 Acknowledgements

The author acknowledges the consultant nurse/midwife team at the Oxford Radcliffe Hospitals NHS Trust for the development of a clear example of a job description that includes non-medical prescribing as a key element of the role, and their agreement to incorporate this as an example of good practice.

1:4 Answers to 'Test your knowledge about the law as it applies to non-medical prescribing' quiz

(1) Professional responsibility in relation to prescribing refers to up to date knowledge of drugs and medicines and their actions; knowledge of the legal framework of drugs and medicines that govern licensing, supply and administration as applicable to the non-medical prescribing role. There is also a requirement to demonstrate competency within all skills that relate to prescribing.

(2) 1968 Medicines Act, 1971 Misuse of Drugs Act.

(3) Supply, storage and administration of medicines.

(4) Medicines Healthcare Regulatory Agency website, BNF, e-cab bulletins.
(5) 1 May 2006.
(6) Standards of Proficiency for Nurse and Midwife Prescribers.
(7) Nurses, Pharmacists, Chiropodists, Podiatrists, Radiographers, Physiotherapists.
(8) Doctors, dentists, vets, the following groups of qualified non-medical prescribers – nurses, pharmacists, optometrists.
(9) National Prescribing Centre (NPC).

APPENDIX 2

Prescribing Practice from the Employer's Perspective: The Rationale for CPD within Non-Medical Prescribing

This appendix relates to Chapter 2 and includes a brief list of web sites that provide resources to support the rationale for CPD in non-medical prescribing, from the organisational perspective. In addition, a clinical governance self-assessment and action planning tool is offered as an example of good practice in monitoring and evaluation of non-medical prescribing practice.

2:1   Useful websites

NHS London Pharmacy Education and Training
   http://www.londonpharmacy.nhs.uk/educationandtrsaining/
   ksf/ksf.aspx
The Association of the British Pharmaceutical Industry
   http://www.abpi.org.uk/

2:2   Example of a clinical governance tool for a health-care organisation to support non-medical prescribing

NHS
London

Non-Medical Prescribing (NMP)
Clinical Governance Self-Assessment and Action Planning Tool

July 2008

This tool is designed to be used to allow an individual health care provider organisation or a commissioning body to be able to asses or stipulate the clinical governance arrangements that should be in place with respect to non-medical prescribing (NMP) to improve safety and reduce clinical risk. It is issued as guidance and may be adapted for local use. It is recommended that the organisation's clinical governance lead or equivalent assess the policies, systems and processes that are in place and provide the organisation with the assurance that non-medical prescribing arrangements are fit for purpose.

It is suggested that while the regulations and guidance related to NMP is being changed and developed, an assessment of local arrangements may be needed every six months. The results may form the basis of annual work plans.

Responsibility for assessment: ....   **Date assessment performed:** ....

                                                      Date for next review: ....

INTRODUCTION

Non-medical prescribing aims to maximise benefits to patients and the NHS by

- Providing better access to and use of medicines;
- Providing better, more flexible use of workforce skills;
- Ensuring that quality and patient safety underpins this provision.

Prescribing rights have been extended to nurses, midwives, pharmacists, physiotherapists, radiographers, chiropodists/ podiatrists and optometrists. It is important that these activities are acknowledged and supported so that they deliver safe, effective, patient care. Updates on future changes can be found on the Department of Health website, http://www.dh.gov.uk/en/Policyandguidance/Medicinespharmacyandindustry/Prescriptions/TheNon-MedicalPrescribingProgramme/index.htm. or, as the site changes regularly, by using a search engine.

Effective Clinical Governance in non-medical prescribing will help to minimise risks by ensuring the utilisation of effective systems with clear lines of accountability and responsibility. A systematic process will ensure the relevant development, training and supervision for our professional staff who are prescribers and will support the delivery of safe and effective treatment for patients

The Health Care Commission's, 'National Standards, Local Action Health and Social Care Standards and Planning Framework' (DH 2005/06-2007/08) has published standards for better health, which should be taken into account by those providing NHS Care directly, those managing the health service and those commissioning healthcare. The Standards are organised into seven domains as follows: Safety, Clinical and Cost Effectiveness, Governance, Patient Focus, Accessible and Responsive Care, Care and Environmental Amenities, Public Health.

Therefore, when we consider Clinical Governance and Health-Care Commission's Standards, and relate them to non-medical prescribing in this assessment tool, we identify that it will provide a number of benefits.

It will help health-care organisations to

- understand their responsibilities in relation to the implementation of non-medical prescribing;
- identify where they are meeting their statutory obligations and where improvement is required;
- prompt the development of an appropriate infrastructure, to support and maintain non-medical prescribing;
- raise awareness of the benefits of non-medical prescribing in the provision of services is and promote interest in utilising non-medical prescribing more widely;
- give assurance to commissioners and organisations of their own safe and effective management of non-medical prescribers;
- give assurance to the patients and public of mechanisms in place for the prescribing of medicines to them.

THE TOOL

1. SAFETY

Patient safety is enhanced by the use of healthcare processes, working practices and systemic activities that prevent or reduce risk of harm to patients

STANDARD	In place	Not in place	Evidence or Action Plan	By whom & by when
1.1 There is a current database of qualified and registered non-medical prescribers (NMPs)				
1.2 The health care organisation maintains a central administrative contact point for any queries on the prescribing status of NMPs				
1.3 Mechanisms exist that identify and learn from all patient safety incidents and other reportable incidents, and make improvements in practise based on local and national experience and information derived from the analysis of incidents				
1.4 Mechanisms exist to ensure all NMPs are kept informed of relevant clinical information, e.g. Patient Safety Notices, Drug Alerts and Hazard Warnings				
1.5 Patient safety notices, alerts and other communications concerning patient safety which require action are acted upon within required timescales				
1.6 There is a system for the acquisition and retention of specimen signatures to identify prescribers				
1.7 There is a system for ordering and receiving and safely storing secure stationery including prescription pads as used in all settings				
1.8 There is a system for retrieving prescription pads for staff leaving (as appropriate)				
1.9 There is a system in place for ordering and distribution of BNFs and the Nurse Prescribers' Formulary for Community Practitioners as appropriate				
1.10 In any setting the mechanisms for supply of medicines should be reviewed so that where possible prescribing and supply/dispensing are separated and appropriate checks are in place				
1.11 Procedures exist to identify and remedy poor performance				

2. CLINICAL AND COST EFFECTIVENESS

Patients achieve healthcare benefits that meet their individual needs through healthcare decisions and services, based on what assessed research evidence has shown provides effective clinical outcomes

STANDARD	In place	Not in place	Evidence or Action Plan	By whom & by when
2.1 Ensure that non-medical prescribers (NMPS) have access to a prescribing budget				
2.2 Systems for monitoring prescribing are in place in all sectors of practice (e.g. PACT data)				
2.3 The health care organisation has local formularies and guidelines to support evidence based, cost effective prescribing				
2.4 Non-medical prescribers are involved in the development of these formularies and guidelines				
2.5 NMPs are receiving appropriate support or supervision in their prescribing role (e.g. local clinical supervision groups/ learning sets or peer-support groups)				
2.6 Standards from Regulatory bodies and National Prescribing Centre Competency Frameworks http://www.npc.co.uk/non_medical/competency_frameworks.htm are used to inform the development of non-medical prescribers				
2.7 NMPs have an agreed scope of practice or equivalent and a copy of this is retained by the organisation				
2.8 NMPs identify and fulfil continuing professional development needs relevant to their clinical work				
2.9 NMPs participate in regular clinical audit and reviews of their clinical services.				
2.10 Prescribing for children is restricted to those who have the relevant training and experience				

3. GOVERNANCE

Managerial and clinical leadership and accountability, as well as the organisation's culture, systems and working practices, ensure that probity, quality assurance, quality improvement and patient safety are central components of all activities of the healthcare organization

STANDARD	In place	Not in place	Evidence or Action Plan	By whom & by when
3.1 There is an up to date non-medical prescribing policy in place				
3.2 There is a policy covering the use of unlicensed medicines, and medicines used outside the terms of their marketing authorisation?				
3.3 There is a Controlled Drug Policy that includes prescribing by non-medical prescribers and that reflects the most recent legislation, regulation and guidance				
3.4 The organisation has a policy for the reporting of adverse events, which is linked into the NPSA national system for reporting and learning http://www.npsa.nhs.uk/ and to the MHRA systems http://www.mhra.gov.uk/home/idcplg?IdcService=SS_GET_PAGE&nodeId=285				
3.5 There is a Service Level Agreement (SLA) or other written agreement for contractors (e.g. pharmacists) and practice staff with the organisation to confirm that prescribing activity will follow organisation guidelines and clinical governance requirements.				
3.6 The organisation has transparent and consistent policies regarding involvement with the Pharmaceutical Industry				
3.7 NMPs have appropriate indemnity arrangements.				
3.8 Employed staff have the non-medical prescribing role included in their contract of employment, job description or other relevant document for the purposes of vicarious liability				
3.9 There are clear lines of responsibility and accountability for overall quality of clinical care				
3.10 NMPs undertake a CRB check as required by local policy				
3.11 Monitor non-medical prescribing legislation and ensure that policies are updated in line with the revised legislation				
3.12 There is a mechanism in place to ensure the selection of suitable candidates for training				
3.13 Pharmacist prescribers do not direct prescriptions they have written to their pharmacy or any other pharmacy in particular				
3.14 NMPs do not prescribe for themselves. Prescribing for anyone with whom they have a close personal relationship should only occur in exceptional circumstances				

4. PATIENT FOCUS

Healthcare is provided in partnership with patients, their carers and relatives, respecting their diverse needs, preferences and choices, and in partnership with other organizations [especially social care organizations] whose services impact on patient well being

STANDARD	In place	Not in place	Evidence or Action Plan	By whom & by when
4.1 Patient Information about Non-Medical Prescribing (NMP) is available in appropriate formats				
4.2 Users are involved in the design and content of the patient information.				
4.3 Patient forums are informed about the development of NMP				
4.4 Systems are in place to monitor patients' experience of non-medical prescribing				
4.5 Non-medical prescribers receive feedback from Public and Patient Involvement Forum or those monitoring the patient experience				

5. ACCESSIBLE AND RESPONSIVE CARE

Patients receive services as promptly as possible, have choice in access to services and treatments, and do not experience unnecessary delay at any stage of service delivery or the care pathway

STANDARD	In place	Not in place	Evidence or Action Plan	By whom & by when
5.1 Consideration has been given to cover for absence and succession planning				
5.2 Non-medical prescribers' access to computer-generated prescriptions and decision making support is supported as required for their role.				

6. CARE ENVIRONMENT AND AMENITIES

Care is provided in environments that promote patient and staff wellbeing and respect for patients' needs and preferences in that they are designed for the effective and safe delivery of treatment, care or a specific function

STANDARD	In place	Not in place	Evidence or Action Plan	By whom & by when
6.1 Health care is provided in an environment which is supportive of patient privacy and confidentiality.				
6.2 Health care must be provided in a safe and secure environment which protects patients, staff, visitors and their property, and the physical assets of the organisation				
6.3 Environments where health care is delivered are well maintained with cleanliness levels in clinical and non clinical areas that meet the national specification for clean NHS premises				

7. PUBLIC HEALTH

Programmes and services are designed and delivered in collaboration with all relevant organizations and communities to promote, protect and improve the health of the population served and reduce health inequalities between different population groups and areas

STANDARD	In place	Not in place	Evidence or Action Plan	By whom & by when
7.1 Health care organisations have systematic and managed disease prevention and health promotion programmes which meet the requirements of the National Service Frameworks and national plans with particular regard to reducing obesity through action on nutrition and exercise, smoking, substance misuse and sexually transmitted infections.				

Documents informing the development of this tool

Supporting documents available on National Electronic Library for Medicines (site is due to be updated shortly)
http://www.nelm.nhs.uk/search/product.aspx?id=71

An Evaluation of Extended Formulary Independent Nurse Prescribing - on the Department of Health website
http://www.dh.gov.uk/PublicationsAndStatistics/Publications/PublicationsPolicyAndGuidance/PublicationsPolicyAndGuidanceArticle/fs/
en?CONTENT_ID=4114084&chk=16BUDW

Nursing and Midwifery Council: Standards of Proficiency for Nurse and Midwife prescribers

Clinical Governance Framework for Pharmacist Supplementary Prescribers

Royal Pharmaceutical Society of Great Britain (Oct. 2005) http://www.rpsgb.org in Clinical Governance section

National Primary and Care Trust Supplementary Prescribing Toolkit **(largely attributable to Shropshire and South Staffordshire Trusts)**

Saving lives: A delivery programme to reduce healthcare associated infection (HCAI) including MRSA – on the Department of Health website

Healthcare Commission- http://www.healthcarecommission.org.uk/homepage.cfm

2:3   Acknowledgements

We are very grateful to Jane Nicholls, NHS London Non-Medical Prescribing Lead, and Marcia Osuno in Barking and Havering PCT, who developed this tool and have given their permission for its use as an illustration of good practice in monitoring and audit of clinical governance in relation to non-medical prescribing.

APPENDIX 3

Writing and Maintaining a Non-Medical Prescribing Policy for Your Organisation

This section contains resources that relate to Chapter 3, in which the importance of developing an organisational policy is stressed. A brief list of useful websites is included, along with an example non-medical prescribing policy that illustrates the suggestions discussed in Chapter 3.

3:1 Useful websites

Clinical Management Plans
http://www.cmponline.info

National Prescribing Centre
http://www.npc.co.uk

Nursing & Midwifery Council
http://www.nmc-uk.org

Pharmacy Post-Graduate education
http://www.cppe.mam.ac.uk

3:2 Example non-medical prescribing policy for a health-care organisation

Contents

1. *Foreword*
2. *Background*
3. *Local Policy*
   3.1   *Patient Group Directions*

1. Foreword

Non-medical prescribing covers both independent and supplementary prescribing by non-medical practitioners (such as nurses and pharmacists). Legislation governs who may prescribe which medicines under which circumstances. This is a rapidly expanding area with regular changes to the prescribing current non-medical prescribers can undertake and the addition of other allied health professions as non-medical prescribers. This policy has been written to include all Department of Health guidance and to inform clinical areas, managers, current non-medical prescribers and potential non-medical prescribers. As each group has more interest in some sections than others, each section has been written to be self-explanatory.

Trust Policy

This document outlines the administrative and procedural steps needed to enable registered nurses, registered midwives and registered pharmacists to act as non-medical prescribers within the Trust, so that practice is within the law, has the approval of the Trust, is compatible with service development plans, benefits patient care and is an appropriate extension of a practitioner's role. It also serves allied health professionals as they become designated to undertake supplementary and/or independent prescribing. In April 2005 legislation allowed physiotherapists, radiographers and chiropodists/podiatrists to train as supplementary prescribers. In August 2007, legislation allowed optometrists to train as supplementary prescribers.

2. Background

Before April 2002, medicines legally designated as Prescription-only Medicines (POMs), could generally only be prescribed by a doctor or dentist. They were also solely responsible for and organised every change to a patient's medication when a POM was involved. Supplementary prescribing has its basis in the recommendations of the final report of the 'Review of Prescribing, Supply and Administration of Medicines' (1999) led by Dr June Crown, which recommended the introduction of a new form of prescribing, to be undertaken by non-medical health professionals after a diagnosis had been made and a clinical management plan had been drawn up for the patient by a doctor. It recommended that two types of prescriber should be recognised:

Independent prescribers, who would be responsible for the assessment of patients with undiagnosed conditions and for decisions about the clinical management required, including prescribing.

Supplementary prescribers (previously referred to as dependent prescribers), who would be responsible for the continuing care of patients who have been clinically assessed by an independent prescriber. This continuing care might include prescribing, which would usually be informed by clinical guidelines and be consistent with individual treatment plans, or continuing established treatments by issuing repeat prescriptions, with the authority to adjust the dose or dosage form according to the patient's needs. The Crown Review recommended that there should be provision for regular clinical review by the assessing clinician.

Following publication of the Crown Report, Health Ministers decided to focus initially on extending nurse prescribing. Extended Formulary Nurse Prescribing (or Independent Nurse Prescribing) was introduced in 2002. The Department of Health and the Medicines Control Agency then undertook a public consultation between April and July 2002 on proposals to implement supplementary prescribing for nurses and pharmacists. Lord Philip Hunt announced plans to introduce supplementary prescribing in November 2002 and the legal changes came into force in April 2003.

Legal basis of non-medical independent and supplementary prescribing – Section 63 of the Health and Social Care Act 2001 allows Ministers, by Order, to designate new categories of prescriber, and to set conditions for their prescribing. Amendments to the 1968 Medicines Act various Prescription-only Medicines Orders and changes to NHS Regulations designate which medicines can be prescribed, by whom and under what circumstances.

3. Local Policy

The Trust recognises that the traditional description of professional relationships among doctors, dentists, nurses and pharmacists no longer fully reflects the needs of modern clinical practice. It is desirable that highly trained health-care professionals should be able to use their full range of skills in the interests of better care, the efficient use of resources and enhanced job satisfaction. This reflects the ethos of the Trust in developing both new roles and new ways of working and supporting service re-design. It is essential, however, that the extension of professional roles is accompanied by clear arrangements for accountability. Extending the role of health-care practitioners must take into account the need to benefit patient care, to ensure continuity of care, to protect patient safety, to safeguard patient choice, to be convenient and cost effective. Arrangements should additionally be considered to backfill previous roles.

There are various mechanisms for prescribing by nurses/midwives, pharmacists and other allied health professionals and for the supply and administration of medicines by a wider range of health care professionals.

3.1 *Patient Group Directions* (PGDs) are not a form of prescribing, but are written instructions for the supply or administration of medicines to groups of patients *who may not be individually identified before presentation for treatment*. The majority of clinical care is still expected to be provided on an individual, patient-specific basis. Consequently the supply and administration of medicines under Patient Group Directions should be reserved for circumstances in which they offer an advantage for patient care (without compromising patient safety), and when they are consistent with appropriate professional relationships and accountability. PGDs do not allow 'prescriptions to be written' to authorise another nurse or health professional to administer medicines. PGDs have a role within secondary care practice and their place in improving service delivery to patients within the Trust may be accessible to a wider range of healthcare professionals than supplementary or independent prescribing.

3.2 *Prescribing by District Nurses and Health Visitors –*   Following training incorporated into their specialist practitioner programmes, district nurse and health visitor independent prescribers can prescribe from the Community Practitioners Formulary for District Nurses and Health Visitors; this can be found at the back of the BNF: it comprises a limited list of medicines and a large number of dressings and appliances relevant to community nursing and health visiting practice.

3.3 *Independent Nurse Prescribers*   undertake a longer, specific programme of preparation and from May 2006 have been allowed to prescribe licensed medicines for any medical condition that a nurse prescriber is competent to treat, including a limited range of controlled drugs. Between 2002 and March 2006 independent nurse prescribers were prescribing from a frequently changing Nurse Pre-scribers Extended Formulary.

3.4 Independent Prescribing by Pharmacists was also introduced in May 2006, but pharmacists currently can only prescribe licensed medicines (excluding controlled drugs) for any medical condition that a pharmacist prescriber is competent to treat.

3.5 Supplementary Prescribing allows appropriately trained and registered nurses, pharmacists and other allied health professionals to prescribe in partnership with an independent medical prescriber, i.e. doctor or dentist. There is no legal restriction on the clinical conditions that may be dealt with by a supplementary prescriber. Although supplementary prescribing is primarily intended for use in managing specific chronic medical conditions or health needs affecting the patient, acute episodes can be treated, provided they are included in the clinical management plan (CMP). Supplementary prescribers can prescribe all medicines. A patient specific CMP is drawn up, with the patient's agreement, following diagnosis of the patient's condition by the independent medical prescriber, and following consultation and agreement between the independent and supplementary prescribers. Time spent initially developing a simple CMP should be time saved when the patient returns for review. Different allied health professions (AHPs) are gradually being approved as supplementary prescribers. In April 2005, legislative changes approved physiotherapists, chiropodists/podiatrists and radiographers and in August 2007, optometrists were added.

Specific examples setting out where non-medical prescribing is of benefit to patients/clients in the local context could be illustrated here.

The Trust therefore supports the appropriate establishment of non-medical prescribing with a view to improving patient care, in particular, access to medication, appropriate and timely treatment, and effective utilisation of the skills of the workforce.

4. Principles of Non-Medical Prescribing

- Patient safety is paramount.
- There must be benefit to patients (e.g. more efficient access to medicines).
- Non-medical prescribing should support, not replace multi-disciplinary care.
- Non-medical prescribing must make best use of the skills of trained nurses, pharmacists and AHPs.

- Non-medical prescribing does not supersede or replace the need for Patient Group Directions when they are more appropriate.
- The patient (or where appropriate their carer/parent) agrees to the arrangement.
- Prescribing and dispensing responsibilities, and prescribing and administration responsibilities should, where possible, be separate in keeping with the principles of patient safety and governance.

5. Framework for Non-Medical Prescribing

5.1 Supplementary Prescribing

(a) Supplementary prescribing is a partnership between the independent and the supplementary prescriber.

(b) Both the independent prescriber and the supplementary prescriber will need preparatory training before entering a prescribing partnership.

(c) The independent prescriber must be a doctor or dentist. It is for the independent prescriber to determine which patients may benefit from supplementary prescribing and the medicines that maybe prescribed by the supplementary prescriber under the clinical management plan (CMP). When coming to a decision, the independent prescriber will need to take account of the professional relationship between the independent and supplementary prescriber as well as the experience and degree of expertise of the supplementary prescriber.

(d) The independent prescriber and the supplementary prescriber must be willing and able to work together. There should be ready lines of communication. They should share access to, consult, and use a common patient record.

(e) The independent prescriber is responsible for diagnosis and for setting the parameters of the CMP, although they need not draw it up themselves.

(f) The CMP can be written or electronic. It relates to a named patient and to that patient's specific condition(s). Agreement to the plan must be recorded by both the independent and supplementary prescriber before supplementary prescribing begins.

(g) In each case the independent and/or supplementary prescriber should obtain the patient's agreement to supplementary prescribing – this need not be written consent. Every effort should be made to obtain informed consent, however, if this is not possible e.g. minors, mental incapacity or unconscious patients, the usual Trust process for consent should be followed.

(h)   Independent and supplementary prescribers must maintain communication on an ad-hoc basis while the supplementary prescriber is reviewing and prescribing for the patient.

(i)   The independent and supplementary prescriber should normally carry out a formal clinical review at the agreed time – normally within 12 months of the start of the CMP. Periods longer than 12 months, between joint clinical reviews or reviews by the independent prescriber, may occasionally be acceptable in the CMP when the patient's condition is stable and deterioration is not to be expected over a period longer than 12 months. The appropriateness of a prolonged review period is the responsibility of the independent prescriber, although it must be agreed with the supplementary prescriber. If joint clinical review is not possible, the outcome of clinical review by the independent prescriber must be discussed with the supplementary prescriber, who must agree continuation of, or changes to, the CMP.

(j)   The independent prescriber should be the clinician or team of clinicians responsible for the individual's care at the time that supplementary prescribing is to start. If this responsibility moves from one independent prescriber to another (for example from the patient's GP to a hospital consultant, or from one GP to another), the supplementary prescriber may not continue to prescribe, unless he/she negotiates and records in the shared patient record a new agreement to enter a prescribing partnership with the new independent prescriber and patient. Supplementary prescribing partnerships can involve more than one independent prescriber.

(k)   The supplementary prescriber is accountable for all decisions made and the prescribing they undertake.

(l)   The supplementary prescriber has discretion in the choice of dosage, frequency, product, and other variables in relation to medicines only within the limits specified by the CMP. The CMP may include reference to authoritative clinical guidelines and guidance (local or national), whether written or electronic, as an alternative to listing medicines individually. Any guidelines referred to should be readily accessible to the supplementary prescriber when managing the patient's care.

5.2 Supplementary Prescribing – Responsibilities of the Independent Medical Prescriber and Supplementary Prescriber

5.2.1 The independent medical prescriber is responsible for:

(a)   The initial clinical assessment of the patient, the formulation of the diagnosis and determining the scope of the CMP.

(b) Reaching an agreement with the supplementary prescriber about the limits of their responsibility for prescribing and review. This should be set out in the CMP.

(c) Providing advice and support to the supplementary prescriber as requested.

(d) Carrying out a review of the patient's progress at appropriate intervals, depending on the nature and stability of a patient's condition.

(e) Sharing the patient's record with the supplementary prescriber.

(f) Reporting adverse incidents according to Trust procedures, which may inform the National Patient Safety Agency (NPSA) via the National Reporting and Learning System; and reporting adverse reactions to the Medicines and Health-care products Regulatory Agency (MHRA).

(g) The independent prescriber may, *at any time*, review the patient's treatment and/or resume full responsibility for the patient's care.

5.2.2 The supplementary prescriber is responsible for:

(a) Prescribing for the patient in accordance with the CMP. Altering the medicines prescribed, within the limits set out in the CMP, if monitoring of the patient's progress indicates that this is clinically appropriate.

(b) Monitoring and assessing the patient's progress as appropriate to the patient's condition and the medicines prescribed.

(c) Working at all times within their clinical competence and their professional Code of Conduct, and consulting the independent prescriber when necessary.

(d) Accepting professional accountability and clinical responsibility for their prescribing practice.

(e) Passing prescribing responsibility to the independent prescriber if the agreed clinical reviews are not carried out within the specified interval or if they feel that the management of the patient's condition no longer falls within their sphere of competence.

(f) Recording prescribing and monitoring activity contemporaneously in the shared patient record, highlighting that the non-medical prescriber is acting as a supplementary prescriber.

5.2.3 Working together

(a) Independent and supplementary prescribers must be willing and able to work together and to assume the specific responsibilities listed above.

(b) Independent and supplementary prescribers may work in more than one prescribing partnership, providing that in each case they work as described above.

5.3 The Clinical Management Plan (CMP)

(a) The Clinical Management Plan (CMP) is the foundation stone of supplementary prescribing and must include the following:

- The name of the patient to whom the plan relates.
- The illness or conditions that may be treated by the supplementary prescriber.
- The date on which the plan is to take effect, and when it is to be reviewed by the doctor or dentist who is party to the plan.
- Refer to the class or description of medicines or appliances that may be prescribed or administered under the CMP. The CMP must include a reference to published national or local guidelines. These must clearly identify the range of relevant medicinal products to be used to treat the patient and the CMP should draw attention to the relevant part(s) of the guideline(s). Any guideline referred to must be easily accessible. The CMP should state the circumstances in which the dose, frequency and formulation can be varied.
- Any restrictions or limitations as to the strength or dose of any medicine that may be prescribed or administered under the plan and any period of administration or use of any medicine or appliance that may be prescribed under the plan or in supporting guidelines.
- Relevant warnings about known sensitivities of the patient to, or known difficulties of the patient with, particular medicines or appliances.
- The arrangements for notification of: -
  - o suspected or known reactions to any medicine that may be prescribed or administered under the plan, and suspected or known adverse reactions to any other medicine taken at the same time as any medicine prescribed or administered under the plan.
  - o incidents occurring with the appliance which might lead, might have led or have led to the death or serious deterioration of the health of the patient.
- The circumstances in which the supplementary prescriber should refer to, or seek the advice of, the doctor or dentist who is party to the plan.

(b) The independent prescriber (IP) must determine how much responsibility he or she wants to give to the supplementary prescriber (SP). This will take account of the experience and skills of the individual SP.

(c) The CMP may be paper-based (e.g. patient held record) or electronic/IT-based and ideally should be simple and quick to complete.

(d) The clinical management plan must be agreed before supplementary prescribing can take place.

(e) The CMP must be included in the patient record.

(f) Nationally agreed sample templates of the clinical management plan may be attached as appendices.

(g) Examples of CMPs developed or in use locally could be offered in a further appendix.

(h) The CMP must be agreed between independent medical prescriber and supplementary prescriber.

(i) The CMP comes to an end:

- at any time at the discretion of the independent prescriber,
- at the request of the supplementary prescriber or the patient,
- at the time specified for the review of the patient (unless it is renewed by both prescribers at that time),
- when there is a sole independent prescriber and he or she is replaced for whatever reason. In these circumstances the CMP must be reviewed by their successor.

5.4 Independent Prescribing – Responsibilities of the Non-Medical Prescriber

Independent non-medical prescribers must only prescribe from the medicines the law allows them to prescribe and only for the medical conditions they are competent to treat. Clear professional guidance is offered for nurse independent prescribers from the Nursing and Midwifery Council (NMC) and pharmacist independent prescribers from the Royal Society of Pharmacists of Great Britain (RSPGB).

5.5 Who May Prescribe?

Appropriately qualified and registered nurses/midwives and pharmacists, and other health-care professionals, as they become eligible, may prescribe.

To be legally eligible to prescribe from the Prescription-only Medicines (POM) Order and NHS Regulations, and to meet the Trust criteria for non-medical prescribing, staff must fulfil all of the following:

5.5.1 Pharmacists

(a) Be a UK registered pharmacist
(b) Have at least 2 years post registration experience.
(c) Have the ability to study at a minimum of QAA level 3, and to have successfully completed the recognised training and assessment for prescribing
(d) Have a mark against their name in the professional register, i.e. record their prescribing competency on the register of the Royal Pharmaceutical Society of Great Britain indicating that they hold this qualification and are trained as supplementary pharmacist prescriber.
(e) Be employed by the Trust and be registered with the Trust as a non-medical prescriber (see section 5.6.3)
(f) Be working in a post in which non-medical prescribing will be beneficial to patient care.
(g) Their job description should reflect that they are a non-medical prescriber.
(h) There are backfill arrangements in place for the duties the non-medical prescriber can no longer undertake as they are now taking on an extended role.

5.5.2 Nurses and midwives

(a) Be a first level UK registered nurse or UK registered midwife.
(b) Have at least 3 years post-registration clinical nursing experience, having spent the year preceding preparation for a prescribing role working in the specialty in which they intend to prescribe
(c) Nurses/midwives will usually be at Band 5 or above
(d) Should have a current CRB check
(e) Have skills in history taking and physical assessment in order to make a diagnosis relevant to the prescribing of medication in the specialty
(f) Have the ability to study at Level 3 (degree level) and have successfully completed the recognised training and assessment for non-medical prescribing.
(g) Have a mark against their name in the Nursing and Midwifery Council (NMC) professional register indicating that they hold this qualification and are trained as supplementary nurse prescriber and/or independent nurse prescriber.
(h) Be employed by the Trust and be registered at the Trust as a non-medical prescriber (see section 5.6.3)
(i) Be working in a post in which non-medical prescribing will be beneficial to patient care.

(j) Their job description should reflect that they are a non-medical prescriber.

(k) There are backfill arrangements in place for the duties the non-medical prescribers can no longer undertake as they are now taking on an extended role.

5.5.3 Allied health professionals

There are similar criteria for registered AHPs, including the ability to study at a minimum of Level 3 and to have at least three years relevant post-qualification experience. Further information is available on the Health Professions Council website http://www.hpc-uk.org.

5.6 Registering as a Non-Medical Prescriber Within the Trust

This section should clearly indicate the process practitioners should follow in order to register their intention to prescribe within the organisation, and direct the reader to a registration from or process that could be included as an appendix

The following criteria must be met to register as a non-medical prescriber at the Trust:

5.6.1 Training

The non-medical prescriber must have successfully completed the appropriate accredited training and preparation for non-medical prescribing, including all assessments and the period of learning in practice.

It is the responsibility of the line manager and the medical supervisor to ensure that the non-medical prescriber has the knowledge and skills to prescribe as a component of their role. The course does not teach clinical knowledge and its application in practice: this is assessed by the medical supervisor during the 12 days of supervised practice.

The National Prescribing Centre (http:// www.npc.org) has produced a guide to help doctors prepare for and carry out the role of designated medical practitioner (supervisor) – it is called Training non-medical prescribers in practice – a guide to help doctors prepare for and carry out the role of designated medical practitioner (February 2005).

5.6.2 Registration with professional body

The non-medical prescriber must ensure that his/her non-medical prescribing competence is registered with his/her relevant professional body.

(a) For *Pharmacists* – once a pharmacist has successfully completed an approved educational programme the RPSGB will be notified via the Higher Education Institution. The pharmacists' professional register will be annotated to indicate that the pharmacist has qualified as a non-medical Prescriber.

Confirmation of a pharmacist's prescriber registration can be obtained by contacting the RPSGB on 020 7572 2322 between 9 a.m. and 5 p.m. Monday to Friday. Registration can also be checked on line at: http://www.rpsgb.org.uk/society.

(b) For *Nurses* – once a nurse/midwife has successfully completed an approved educational programme, the Nursing and Midwifery Council UK will be notified via the Higher Education Institution. The NMC professional register will be annotated to indicate that a nurse/midwife has qualified as a prescriber. Confirmation of a nurse's/midwife's prescriber registration can be obtained by contacting the 24 hour NMC confirmation interactive voice response system on Tel: 020 7631 3200.

(c) For *AHPs* – the Health Professions Council has a similar process. Confirmation of an AHP's prescriber registration can be obtained by contacting the Health Professions Council on 0845 300 4472. Registration can also be checked on-line at http://www.hpc-uk.org/register.

5.6.3 Registering with the Trust Non-Medical Prescribers' Register

This section will be individual to an organisation but should specify how the organisation will be notified of a practitioner's intention to prescribe, and where a record of non-medical prescribers will be kept within the organisation. In the acute sector, this record might be held with non-medical prescribing leads, or with the pharmacy department. However in primary care organisations it may be that a practice manager will keep a record, or a record may be held by the prescribing lead for the PCT. The practitioner's professional manager should keep a record for HR purposes.

5.6.4 Maintaining competence to prescribe

(a) All nurses, pharmacists and AHPs have a professional responsibility to keep themselves abreast of clinical and professional developments. Non-medical prescribers are expected to keep up to date with best practice in the management of the conditions for which they prescribe, and in the use of the relevant medicines, dressings and appliances.

(b) The organisation has a responsibility to make available opportunities for continuing professional development (CPD) for non-medical prescribers. This is provided through a combination of seminars and meetings provided at both an organisational and directorate level.

(c)   Non-medical prescribers who change their clinical specialty or join the Trust are advised to undergo a further period of supervised practice before demonstrating to a senior medical clinician their competence to prescribe within that clinical specialty. They should then follow the specified process for registering their intention to prescribe within their specialty (see section 5.6.3).

(d)   Non-medical prescribers who join the Trust working in the same specialty, must ensure they are familiar with Trust policies and procedures relating to prescribing, any treatment guidelines used within their specialty and the Trust Formulary. This could include a period of supervised practice. They should then follow the specified process for registering their intention to prescribe within their specialty (see section 5.6.3).

(e)   Following an extended period of absence (more than six months), such as maternity leave, a career break or secondment to a post without prescribing responsibilities, the non-medical prescriber should work with a senior clinician to ensure that they have retained or regain the competence and confidence to prescribe. They should then follow the specified process for registering their intention to prescribe within their specialty (see section 5.6.3).

(f)   Any change in personal circumstances, for example change of name, should be registered with the non-medical prescribing lead for the organisation.

5.7   For Whom Can Supplementary Prescribers Prescribe?

Supplementary prescribers are allowed to manage patients, with agreed medical conditions, under the care of medical independent prescribers within the Trust, whom the medical independent prescriber has assessed, and to prescribe medicines according to an agreed clinical management plan. The clinical management plan must be agreed between the supplementary prescriber and the medical independent prescriber before they start to prescribe. The patient must also give their consent.

5.8   What May Be Prescribed by Supplementary Prescribers?

Provided medicines are prescribable on the NHS and are referred to in the patient's clinical management plan, supplementary prescribers may prescribe:

- All General Sales List (GSL) medicines,
- Pharmacy (P) medicines,

- Appliances and devices, foods and other borderline substances approved by the Advisory Committee on Borderline
  Substances,
- All Prescription-only Medicines (POMs) licensed for use in the
  UK including "off label" use. For nurses and pharmacists this
  includes controlled drugs specified in the clinical management
  plan,
- Prescription-only Medicines (POMs) that are unlicensed in
  the UK or are "'Specials'", as stated in the clinical management plan provided that prescribing is in accordance
  with the Trust's Policy for Unlicensed Medicines and an unlicensed medicines request form has been completed for the
  patient.

Note: Supplementary prescribers should not agree to prescribe any
medicine if they feel that their knowledge of the medicine falls outside
of their area of competence.

5.9 For Whom and What Can Independent Nurse Prescribers Pre-
scribe?

The independent non-medical prescriber may prescribe for any patient
of any doctor for whom the non-medical prescriber is providing care
and has assessed, who presents with a medical condition that is within
the competency of the prescriber to treat.
What may be prescriber?

- any GSL, P medicines,
- any licensed Prescription-only Medicine
- Nurse independent prescribers may prescribe specified controlled drugs from the list agreed for the Nurse Prescribers
  Extended Formulary.

5.10 Prescribing Paperwork for Non-Medical Prescribers

(a) Non-medical prescribers must use the existing Trust pre-
    scribing paperwork to maintain a contemporaneous record
    of the medication history.
(b) Non-medical prescribers must follow Trust guidelines for
    good prescribing practice.
(c) All Trust prescriptions, i.e. outpatient, day case, discharge
    (TTO) prescriptions forms and in-patient drug charts should
    be marked by the non-medical prescriber's signature with:
    'SNP' for supplementary nurse and midwife prescribers,
    'SPP' for supplementary pharmacist prescribers,
    'INP' for independent nurse prescribers,
    'IPP' for independent pharmacist prescribers,

'SAHP' for supplementary allied health profession prescribers,

to allow easy identification by pharmacists, medical and
nursing staff.

(d) Non-medical prescribers who are required to use FP10 prescriptions to fulfil their role must use the following procedure
in order to obtain FP10 prescriptions.

5.10.1 Ordering of FP10 prescription pads

*This section will be specific to the circumstances of the organisa-
tion, and should relate specifically to the process*

5.10.2 Re-ordering of prescription pads

*This section will be specific to the circumstances of the organisa-
tion, and should relate specifically to the process*

5.10.3 Procedure when a non-medical prescriber leaves the ORH Trust or changes area of clinical practice

(a) It is the responsibility of the nurse's employer, or the chief
pharmacist in the case of a pharmacist, to ensure that no
further FP10HPs are ordered for a non-medical prescriber
who has left employment or been suspended from prescribing duties and to recover and record all unused prescription
forms issued.

(b) On termination of employment, prescription pads must be
returned to the relevant line manager.

(c) Non-medical prescribers' details will be removed from the
pharmacy-held register.

(d) Non-medical prescribers who transfer to a different clinical
area within the Trust must surrender their current pads and
request new FP10HPs to ensure appropriate budgetary management. These can only be used once a period of supervised practice in the new clinical area has been completed
and the non-medical prescriber informs the organisation of
their intention to prescribe.

5.11 Records to Be Kept by Non-Medical Prescribers

(a) All supplementary prescribers must have a valid clinical
management plan for the patient.

(b) All non-medical prescribers are required to keep contemporaneous records, in line with Trust standards for record
keeping and for nurses, guidance from the NMC.

(c) As for medical prescribers a record of the non-medical
prescriber's prescription should be entered into the shared
patient record at the time of writing.

5.12 Administration of Medicines Against Prescriptions from Non-Medical Prescribers

(a) For the administration of medicines, prescriptions of non-medical prescribers should be treated in the same way as prescriptions of doctors and dentists.

(b) All Trust prescriptions, i.e. out-patient, day case, discharge (TTO) prescription forms and in-patient drug charts should be marked by the non-medical prescribers signature with:

'SNP' for supplementary nurse and midwife prescribers,

'SPP' for supplementary pharmacist prescribers

'INP' for independent nurse prescribers

'IPP' for independent pharmacist prescribers,

'SAHP' for supplementary allied health profession prescribers.

to allow easy identification by pharmacists, medical and nursing staff.

(c) Items prescribed by nurse non-medical prescribers should, when possible, be administered by another team member i.e. another appropriately qualified healthcare professional, in keeping with the principles of patient safety and governance. Where this would create an unnecessary delay in the treatment of the patient, the nurse/AHP non-medical prescriber should administer from his/her own prescription following all safety checks to ensure that the patient receives the right medicine, in the right dose and formulation and by the right method of administration.

5.13 Dispensing or Supplying Against Prescriptions from Non-Medical Prescribers

(a) For the dispensing or supply of medicines prescribed by non-medical prescribers, the prescriptions should be treated as for prescriptions from medical prescribers.

(b) All Trust prescriptions, i.e. out-patient, day case, discharge (TTO) prescription forms and in-patient drug charts should be marked by the non-medical prescriber's signature with:

'SNP' for supplementary nurse and midwife prescribers

'SPP' for supplementary pharmacist prescribers

'INP' for independent nurse prescribers

'IPP' for independent pharmacist prescribers

'SAHP' for supplementary allied health profession prescriber

to allow easy identification by pharmacists, medical and nursing staff.

(c) Pharmacy staff should check the prescriber against an up to date register of all qualified non-medical prescribers employed by the Trust and kept in the hospital pharmacy. The same process will apply for all prescriptions.

(d) Prescribing, supply and dispensing responsibilities should, when possible, be separate, in keeping with the principles of patient safety and governance.

(e) Nurses and midwives may be able to *supply* an appropriately pre-packed medicine from pharmacy against the prescription of a non-medical prescriber where such schemes have been set up with the appropriate training.

(f) Items prescribed by a pharmacist non-medical prescriber should preferably be clinically screened by another pharmacist i.e. a pharmacist non-medical prescriber should not *dispense* a prescription that he or she has written, unless in an emergency or when there would be an unacceptable delay to the treatment of a patient. The pharmacist non-medical prescriber must follow all safety checks to ensure that the patient receives the right medicine, in the right dose and formulation and by the right method of administration.

5.14 Security and Safe Handling of Prescriptions by Non-Medical Prescribers

(a) Outpatient, day case, discharge (TTO) prescriptions forms, in-patient drug charts and FP10HP prescriptions are the property of the Trust.

(b) FP10HP prescriptions, in particular, are a target for theft, and the security of all the above prescriptions, when in their possession, rests with prescribers.

(c) An out-patient prescription must only be written/issued when needed and should never be left unattended.

(d) Blank prescriptions must never be pre-signed.

(e) Any concerns relating to the suitability of security arrangements for prescriptions must be brought to the attention of the appropriate manager.

(f) In the event of loss or suspected theft of FP10HP prescriptions the non-medical prescriber must follow the Trust's Handling of FP10s policy.

(g) For electronic prescribing, the non-medical prescriber must keep their password confidential, and when using a terminal should log off immediately after use.

5.15 Reporting Adverse Drug Reactions by Non-Medical Prescribers

(a) If a patient has an adverse reaction to a medicine, the non-medical prescriber must inform the patient's consultant. The incident must be recorded in the patient's hospital notes.

(b) If a patient suffers harm due to an adverse incident involving a medication, or if harm could have been caused to the patient (a near miss), the incident or near miss should be reported by the non-medical prescriber using the Trust incident reporting form, which may feed into the National Patient Safety Agency (NPSA) national reporting system.

(c) The consultant or non-medical prescriber should where appropriate report the adverse incident to the Medicines and Health-care Products Regulatory Agency (MHRA) using the 'yellow card' scheme for reporting adverse drug reactions. (Copies of the 'yellow cards' can be found in the back of the BNF or can be reported on-line).

5.16 Reporting of Prescribing Errors/Near Misses

(a) In instances of errors/near misses the non-medical prescriber must complete the Trust's incident reporting form.

(b) The non-medical prescriber should record the incident in their reflective log and use the event to identify any continuing professional development needs – see sections 5.18 and 8.

5.17 Annual Review by Independent Medical Prescribers of Patients Under the Care of Supplementary Prescribers

Each patient under the care of a supplementary prescriber must be reviewed at least annually by the independent medical prescriber.

5.18 Continuing Education for Non-Medical Prescribers

(a) The Trust supports the National Prescribing Centre's documents and online competency frameworks, and the use of these frameworks in maintaining competence. These can be found on the National Prescribing Centre website:

Http:// www.npc.co.uk/non_medical/competency_ frameworks.htm

(b) Continuing Professional Development (CPD): All prescribers have a professional responsibility to keep themselves abreast of clinical and professional developments. Non-medical prescribers will be expected to keep up to date with best practice in the management of conditions for which they may prescribe, and in the use of the relevant medicines, dressings and appliances.

- Nurses may use the learning from this activity as part of their Post Registration Education and Practice (PREP-CPD) activities.

- For pharmacists it will contribute to the RPSGB's CPD requirements. The curriculum for pharmacists states that pharmacists who register as non-medical prescribers will need to demonstrate evidence of relevant CPD to ensure that their prescribing skills are kept up to date and are extended as their prescribing role develops.
- AHP registrants are required to meet the requirements of the standards of continuing professional development of the HPC. This involves a declaration that they have kept up to date with practice within their current context and scope of practice. It will be subject to periodic audit, requiring the registrant to submit evidence of their CPD to the HPC for scrutiny to support their claim.

(c) It is the responsibility of non-medical prescribers to ensure that they inform their line manager if they feel that their competence or confidence in their prescribing abilities is no longer acceptable or safe. Non-medical prescribers must not prescribe until their needs have been addressed and competence and confidence restored.

(d) The Trust requires non-medical prescribers to maintain a prescribing element in their portfolio of continuing professional development. CPD for the practitioner's role as non-medical prescriber should be included as part of the appraisal process.

(e) Non-medical prescribers must identify their individual training needs with their line manager. These should be included in their personal development plans and linked to appropriate KSFs.

(f) It is the responsibility of the non-medical prescribers to ensure that they remain up to date on therapeutics in the field of their prescribing practice and on changes in national and local prescribing policy. For non-medical prescribers changing their area of practice, the Trust requires a period of supervised practice before registering with the Trust – see section 5.6.3

(g) Non-medical prescribers are encouraged to participate in the Trust's NMP CPD

(h) Department of Health commissioned CPD support is available through the National Prescribing Centre (http://www.npc.co.uk).

(i) For pharmacists the Centre for Pharmacy Post-Graduate Education (http://www.cppe.mam.ac.uk) offers programmes that may be relevant to pharmacist non-medical prescribers.

(j) Use of the RPSGB's clinical governance framework for pharmacist non-medical prescribers is encouraged for both individuals and the organisation and can be found at: http://www.rpsgb.org.uk/pdfs/clincgovframeworkpharm.pdf.

(k)   The Nursing and Midwifery Council published standards of proficiency for nurse/midwife prescribers in 2006 which are available at http:// www.nmc-uk.org.

(l)   Support from other professional colleagues is invaluable to non-medical prescribers, especially those who are newly qualified. Support from a buddy/mentor is to be encouraged. The Trust's Non-Medical Prescribing Leads are able to identify buddy/mentors.

(m)   British National Formularies for Nurse and AHPs NMPs are available through the Deputy Chief Nurse and for pharmacists through the ORH Pharmacy Medicines Information department.

5.19 Working with the Pharmaceutical Industry

(a)   Non-medical prescribers must follow Trust guidelines on working with pharmaceutical industry representatives.

(b)   Non-medical prescribers must follow the Trust 'Conflict of Interest Policy'.

(c)   Non-medical prescribers must follow the Trust and the Department of Health Guidelines on acceptance of gifts and benefits by prescribers issued in November 2003.

(d)   An extract from the Department of Health website reads

'The advertising and promotion of medicines is strictly regulated under the Medicines (Advertising) Regulations of 1994, and it is important that nurse and supplementary prescribers, and indeed all health professionals, make their choice of medicinal product for their patients based on the basis of clinical suitability and value for money alone.

As part of the promotion of a medicine or medicines, suppliers may provide inexpensive gifts and benefits, for example pens, diaries or mouse mats. Personal gifts are prohibited, and it is an offence to solicit or accept a prohibited gift or inducement.

Companies may also offer hospitality at a professional or scientific meeting or at meetings held to promote medicines, but such hospitality should be reasonable in level and subordinate to the main purpose of the meeting.

The Medicines and Health-care products Regulatory Agency (MHRA) is responsible for enforcing the legislation on advertising and promotion of medicines. Any complaints about promotional practices should be referred to the MHRA or to

the industry self regulatory body, the Prescription Medicines Code of Practice Authority.'

5.20 Legal and Clinical Liability

5.20.1 Liability of the employer

Where a non-medical prescriber is appropriately trained and qualified and prescribes as part of their professional duties with the consent of their employer, the employer is held vicariously liable for their actions. In addition:

- Nurse non-medical prescribers are individually professionally accountable to the Nursing and Midwifery Council (NMC) for this aspect of their service, as for any other, and must act at all time in accordance with the NMC Code of Professional Conduct.
- Pharmacist non-medical prescribers are individually professionally accountable to the RSPGB and must at all times act in accordance with the RPSGB Code of Ethics and Standards.
- AHP supplementary prescribers are individually professionally accountable to the Health Professions Council (HPC) and must at all times act in accordance with the HPC's standards of conduct, performance and ethics.

Both the employer and the employee should ensure the employee's job description includes a clear statement that prescribing is required as part of the duties of that post.

5.20.2 Liabilities of the employee

(a) The role of non-medical prescribing must appear in the prescriber's job description.

(b) The non-medical prescriber must be registered with the Trust to prescribe.

(c) The non-medical prescriber must work within the legal framework of the role, within Trust policies, and for supplementary prescribers within the CMP.

5.20.3 Professional indemnity

All non-medical prescribers are advised to have professional indemnity insurance, for instance by means of membership of a professional organisation or trade union or through a personal professional indemnity insurance policy.

5.20.4 Failure to comply with policies

Failure to comply with the Trust's prescribing policies may result in disciplinary action in line with the Trust Performance and Conduct Policy.

6. Role of the Organisation in Non-Medical Prescribing

(a) The Trust as the employer, through the Clinical Directorates will support posts –
  - when there is a patient benefit and an opportunity to act as a non-medical prescriber;
  - by ensuring access to continuing professional development (CPD) opportunities in relation to non-medical prescribing.

(b) Clinical Directorates are expected to:
  - Explore areas where non-medical prescribing can be implemented to benefit patient care.
  - Include non-medical prescribing in Directorate plans, business cases etc.
  - Identify personnel within their area who could undertake non-medical prescribing to benefit patient care.
  - Plan to support the appropriate development of non-medical prescribing, including ensuring that systems are in place to deal with cover/service delivery during periods of both planned absences (e.g. annual leave, study leave) and unplanned absences (e.g. sickness) of the non-medical prescriber and for succession planning.
  - Consider, and plan, how applicants for non-medical prescribing courses will be supported during their training, including cover for study leave, how successful candidates will operate once qualified, and making backfill arrangements for tasks the non-medical prescriber can no longer undertake because of their expanding role.
  - Help identify independent medical prescribers to supervise the training of non-medical prescribers.
  - Make line managers aware that it is their responsibility to ensure that staff operating as non-medical prescribers have read and adhere to this policy.

(c) Clinical Governance Arrangements
  The organisation will follow the clinical governance framework recommended by the Department of Health (*Independent Prescribing Implementation; Department of Health 2006*) and an annual audit of non-medical prescribing will be undertaken by the non-medical prescribing leads. The governance framework includes:
  - Selection criteria for trainees that indicates their potential to prescribe safely.
  - Support for trainees whilst training.
  - Ensuring prescribers are registered with their professional body as a prescriber.

- Ensuring audit, clinical supervision and CPD arrangements are in place.
- Developing a risk management plan
- Ensuring the parameters of an individuals prescribing are agreed between the prescriber, their manager or local professional lead and their employer
- Ensuring the local drug and therapeutics committees are aware of medicines being prescribed.

Selection of Trainees

Potential trainees should contact a Non-Medical Prescribing Lead in order to discuss their role and in order to confirm that they meet both the professional and organisational requirements for entry to the programme, before applying for a course. They should complete a local application form in order to register their interest in becoming a non-medical prescriber before the HEI accepts registration. As a part of this process Potential trainees must:

- Demonstrate evidence of appropriate specialist knowledge
- Demonstrate that they will have the opportunity to prescribe in the post they will occupy on completion of training
- Identify the therapeutic area in advance of training (and in which they hold considerable expertise)
- Be competent to prescribe in the chosen area
- Have the support of their employer
- Demonstrate that their role as a prescriber will meet local service and patient needs
- Ensure any necessary steps to resolve any conflicts of interest that may subsequently arise, where pharmaceutical or other companies have directly or indirectly funded post holders wishing to undertake a programme of preparation to become a prescriber

The Line Manager must confirm:

- The need and the opportunity to act as an NMP immediately on qualifying
- Their agreement about the therapeutic area in which they will prescribe prior to NHS funded training
- Access to a budget for prescribing
- A robust clinical governance framework within which to work
- Support during training and some flexibility for self directed study
- That the post holder has 3 years post qualification experience for nurses, 2 years practice in a clinical environment post registration for pharmacists and AHPS

Non-Medical Prescribing Leads will give priority to:

- Ensuring patient safety
- Maximising benefit to patients and the NHS in terms of quicker and more efficient access to medicines for patients
- Better use of the practitioner's skills
- Informing successful applicants and their line managers in a timely manner.

7. Role of Named Committees, Non-Medical Prescribing Leads and the Pharmacy Department in Non-Medical Prescribing

This section will be specific to the organisation but should specify the role of organisational, nursing and pharmacy committees and the non-medical prescribing designated lead(s) in relation to the process, management and monitoring of non-medical prescribing across the organisation. Importantly this should include who will take responsibility for provision and monitoring of arrangements for CPD.

8. Monitoring and Follow-up of Non-Medical Prescribing

Professional or line managers of non-medical prescribers are expected to review non-medical prescribing from time to time, e.g. as part of the appraisal process. The non-medical prescriber should provide evidence that their role and function are appropriate. The types of issues to be reviewed may include:

- What non-medical prescribers are prescribing and how often.
- What benefits the non-medical prescribing scheme has achieved for patients and how these are reviewed.
- What problems there have been with the implementation and delivery of the scheme, e.g. cover for holidays or succession planning may not have been allowed for; whether peer review schemes for the non-medical prescriber to feedback their prescribing experiences have helped.
- What the effect may have been on local primary care colleagues.
- Use of reflective logs and identification of training needs tools to support CPD.

9. Useful Contact Details

Should include contact details of the Non-Medical Prescribing Leads, and the names of those responsible for drawing up the Policy. It may include contact information from local training opportunities, and for professional organisations for those wishing to confirm registration of non-medical prescribers.

3:3   Acknowledgments

This example policy has been based on a policy developed by current and former Non-Medical Prescribing Leads at the Oxford Radcliffe Hospitals NHS Trust. We are grateful to Jane Hough, Deputy Chief Pharmacist, and the joint Non-Medical Prescribing Lead for permission to base this example on a draft of their policy.

APPENDIX 4

Organising CPD for Non-Medical Prescribers at a Regional Level

This appendix contains a list of websites that relate to organisation of CPD at a regional level, and offers some practical advice from Fiona Peniston-Bird in relation to organisation and facilitation of group learning.

4:1 Useful websites

Department of Health non-medical prescribing homepage
http://www.dh.gov.uk/en/Healthcare/
Medicinespharmacyandindustry/Prescriptions/
TheNon-MedicalPrescribingProgramme/index.htm
Non-medical prescribing CPD Consultancy
http://www.nmprescribing.co.uk/

4:2 How to organise group work for a non-medical prescribing CPD event

- Agree on one issue for discussion.
- Describe the following:
  - What are the key concerns related to this issue?
  - How many within the group have experienced the same issue?
  - What have you tried so far to address it?
  - What would the ideal outcome be?
  - Who would help you reach this outcome?
  - What/who is hindering progression?

- o What are your ideas to reach a solution?
- o Has anyone within the group already found a solution?
- o What is the ideal solution?
- Write your answers onto the flipchart.
- If you finish one issue and have time to discuss more, go ahead!

4:3 How to facilitate a networking session for a non-medical prescribing CPD event

- Organise delegates into groups of 6 + and provide with the following resources, need flip chart paper and pen.
- Ice breaker – invite group participants to introduce each other.
- Invite participants to share the issue that they have brought with them to the event. If they have not brought anything, help them to identify an issue in practice, or if another group has more than one ask if another group can use their issue (if relevant).
- Invite participants to thought shower – using a handout.
- The facilitator moves between the groups helping them as necessary.
- It is the choice of the groups and you if you wish to come together at the end to share the issues and any solutions or action plans.
- Gather up all the flip chart work and summarise, and forward this to participants following the event.

4:4 Acknowledgements

We are grateful to Fiona Peniston-Bird for the practical advice in organising and facilitating group work for non-medical prescribers.

APPENDIX 5

Using E-learning for CPD within Non-Medical Prescribing

In the spirit of the chapter to which it relates, this appendix offers a list of useful websites annotated by Marion Waite, with further details that relate to their usefulness as resources for continuing professional development for non-medical prescribers. In addition, Marion includes the JISC Effective E-learning Planner, which is referred to in Chapter 5.

5:1   Useful websites

BMJ Learning online CPD modules for Doctors, Nurses, Practice Managers, GP Registrars and other health-care professionals – subscription required.
http://learning.bmj.com/learning/main.html

GP Notebook is an online encyclopedia of medicine that provides a trusted immediate reference resource for clinicians in the UK and internationally.
http://www.gpnotebook.co.uk/homepage.cfm

Onmedica is an online resource which is aimed at doctors, nurses, pharmacists, practice managers and health-care students. Onmedica consists of learning modules, journal articles and blogs and is updated on a daily basis. It is free for all health-care staff who possess professional registration.
http://www.onmedica.com/

Intute is a free online resource, which contains quality resources, which have been evaluated by subject specialists for education and research.

Contains a virtual training suite for nurses, midwives and allied health professionals.

http://www.intute.ac.uk/

Rapid e-learning is an online resource, which provides lots of tips about developing and building effective e-learning resources.

http://www.articulate.com/rapid-elearning/

5:2   JISC Effective E-learning Planner

Issues to consider	Designing a learning activity to incorporate ILT or e-learning
1. Learners (their needs, motives for learning, prior experience of learning, social and interpersonal skills, preferred learning styles and ICT competence).	
2. Intended learning outcome (acquisition of knowledge, academic and social skills, increased motivation and ability to progress).	
3. Learning environment (face to face or virtual) – available resources, tools, facilities and services and their match with the learners' needs.	Where does the activity take place?
	What resources are available?
	What technologies are available?
	What features of established practice will be important?
	What support will you require?
4. The learning activity (the means by which the practitioner brings about learning and seeks to influence the development of the learners).	Describe the learning activity

5. The approach taken (related to learners' needs, preferred learning styles, the nature of the learning environment and the intended outcomes).	**Learning styles**
	Inclusion
	Assessment
	ILT or E-learning in Practice
6. How would you evaluate the effectiveness of this learning activity?	**Does this activity engage learners in the learning process?**
	Does this activity encourage independent learning skills?
	Does this activity develop learners' skills and knowledge?
	Does this activity motivate further learning? **ILT or E-learning in Practice**

5:3   Acknowledgements

We are grateful to Sarah Knight, Programme Manager, JISC E-learning Programme, for permission to reproduce the JISC E-learning Planner.

APPENDIX 6

Action Learning
and Learning Sets

This appendix contains a variety of resources that demonstrate examples of good practice. Appendix 6.1 is a tool developed by Yorkshire and the Humber Strategic Health Authority that summarises the excellent work of non-medical prescribers in achieving key organisational and policy outcomes. In Chapter 6 there is a discussion relating to action learning, and a further appendix illustrates the use of a brief case study to facilitate action learning. Key to the acute care context is the high turnover of staff, in particular medical staff, and keeping up to date with medicines management policy in a large organisation is a complex communication issue. Two examples are provided that demonstrate good organisational practice in keeping prescribers abreast of clinical developments, in the form of Medicines Information Leaflets reproduced with the kind permission of the authors.

Action Learning and Learning Sets

DEPARTMENT OF HEALTH

GATEWAY REFERENCE 11538

6:1 Making the connections – using healthcare professionals as prescribers to deliver organisational improvements

There are opportunities for trained non-medical prescribers – nurse and pharmacist prescribers, and other healthcare professionals who have trained as supplementary prescribers (physiotherapists, chiropodist/podiatrists, radiographers and optometrists) to work in parallel with doctors to increase access, capacity and choice for patients.

Policy and Publication Connection examples	How to Use Non-Medical Prescribers in Service Delivery examples	Overarching Key Organisational Benefits
Emergency Care, Urgent and Out of Hours Services	A&E nurse and pharmacist prescribers increase the speed of treating minor illness cases to improve four hour waiting targets, and also allow doctors to concentrate on more complex cases	Financial • reducing doctors' time input • meeting EWTD for junior doctors • increased skill mix, using nurse, pharmacist and other health-care prescribers • reducing drug spend and wastage • reducing staff time and duplicated effort to produce a prescription • preventing admission to hospital • preventing secondary care referrals • managing patients in a community setting • allowing early discharge to intermediate care • avoiding unnecessary delays in discharge
Reforming Emergency Care: First Steps to a New Approach 2001	Community pharmacists prescribing for minor ailments reduce A&E attendance and unnecessary GP visits	
HSC 2003/001 Protecting Staff: delivering services: implementing the European Working Time Directive for doctors in Training	Walk-in Centre nurses offer treatment provision avoiding repeat attendance or a GP visit to obtain a prescription	
Modern Matrons: Improving the Patient's Experience 2003	Nurse practitioners and pharmacists involved in unscheduled care prevent unnecessary hospital admission through work in nursing homes, palliative care and out of hours services	
Creating a Patient Led NHS-Delivering the NHS Improvement Plan 2005	Nurse practitioners can increase access for support and symptom palliation, in terminal care cases	
Practice Based Commissioning: Practical Implementation 2006	Nurse and pharmacist prescribers in substance misuse and rapid access services improve patient access and provide continuity of care, including cover for doctors	

	Use of nurses for chest pain assessment helps reduce admission to hospitals	• meeting QOF and NSF targets for care
	Community pharmacists run travel clinics, enabling GPs to spend more time on more complex cases.	
Delivering the 18 week patient pathway	Community heart failure nurse or pharmacist specialists initiate and titrate medication, provides faster access to treatment, reduce consultant input and readmission to hospital	• adhering to local and national treatment guidelines, containing prescribing costs
Tackling hospital waiting: The 18 week patient pathway. An Implementation Framework 2006	Physiotherapist Supplementary Prescribers for orthopaedics reduce secondary care referrals, orthopaedic consultant input and contribute to meeting the 18 week targets	• reducing prescribing error rates and risks of prescribing errors • Patient Access and Choice • improving patient care through quicker access to medicines
10 High Impact Changes for service improvement and delivery 2004	Pharmacist prescribers help increase the speed of admission and discharge e.g. following surgery	• increasing patient access by service reconfiguration • plurality of provision
National Patient Safety Agency (NPSA) guidance implementation	Tissue viability community services moved from secondary care and developed to reduce patient waits and help achieve 18 week targets	• patient choice about who, when and where services can be accessed
	Pharmacists and nurses prescribers in anticoagulation treat deep vein thrombosis and pulmonary emboli, reducing hospital admissions or length of stay	• local care provision without secondary care visits • providing services in areas where doctors are hard to recruit
	Pharmacist prescribers optimise antimicrobial use, to reduce the incidence of MRSA and clostridium difficile and reduce length of stay.	• allowing doctors time to deal more effectively with complex cases
Increasing Capacity and Efficiency	Family planning services use nurse prescribers to reduce teenage pregnancies	• reducing waiting time for treatment or review • Preventing additional waiting time for patients to see a doctor to get a prescription
The NHS in England: the Operating Framework for 2007\(08 – Dec 2006	Nurse and pharmacist prescribers for contraception and sexual health services improve access and reduce waiting times	

Policy and Publication Connection examples	How to Use Non-Medical Prescribers in Service Delivery examples	Overarching Key Organisational Benefits
Delivering Quality and Value Focus on: productivity and efficiency 2006	Paediatric nurse practitioners and pain management specialists improve timely prescribing, avoid unnecessary delays in treatment and facilitate early discharge	Financial Patient Access and Choice (previously listed)
HSC 2003/001 Protecting Staff: delivering services: implementing the European Working Time Directive for doctors in Training High Impact Changes for practice teams 2006 Choosing Health: Making healthy choices easier 2004	Neonatal nurse practitioner roles developed in line with EWTD, with skills developed to operate at SHO level	
The NHS Plan: a plan for investment, a plan for reform 2000 and Liberating the talents: Helping PCTs and nurses to deliver the NHS Plan 2002	Pharmacist prescribers run clinics for hepatitis B, which promotes adherence to treatment regimes and the uptake of screening. This helps reduce disease progression and transmission, by increasing awareness and understanding amongst patients, their families and communities	
Supporting Long Term Conditions, reducing admissions, hospital stay and delayed discharge	Community Matrons as prescribers improve service access and help prevent avoidable admissions	
Supporting People with Long Term Conditions 2005	Practice nurses and pharmacists for diabetes services, hypertension and hyperlipidaemia reduce GP waiting times, improve patient access to services, increase prescription review and reduce drug wastage. All patients are monitored in line with Diabetes NSF – which was previously more ad hoc	

Implementing Care Closer to Home: Convenient Quality Care for Patients 2007	Physiotherapist Supplementary Prescribers prescribing for patients with respiratory conditions, reducing COPD admissions and enabling earlier discharge
Our Health, Our Care, Our Say: A new direction for community services 2006	Podiatrist supplementary prescribing for diabetic patients enables faster access to treatment, avoids a separate GP visit to get a prescription, improves patient concordance
Practice Based Commissioning: Practical Implementation 2006	Nurse and Pharmacist prescribers for renal patients reduce doctors hours, adhere to local and national guidance, identify medication errors and save costs by reducing drug wastage
The NHS Improvement Plan 2004	Physiotherapist Supplementary Prescribers in intermediate care admit and discharge patients. Reduces use of call-out service for a doctor to prescribe, saves time and money, while also improving concordance
NSFs e.g. Diabetes 2001, Renal 2004/05, Long term Conditions 2005	Intermediate care nurse practitioners and pharmacist prescribers reduce the length of hospital stay and the need for medical input in continuing care
	Nurse and Pharmacist prescribers in nursing homes and mental health services optimise prescribing and reduce drug wastage
	Pharmacist prescribers in cardiovascular/heart failure clinics optimise treatment to increase quality of life, improve QOF target achievement, reduce admissions

6:2   Acknowledgements

We are grateful to the Department of Health and in particular, to Stuart Merritt, for permission to reproduce the document 'Making the Connections', taken from the DH website. This work was led by Yorkshire and Humberside SHA, with contributions from the Department of Health. This represents a particularly good example of how service improvements incorporating non-medical prescribing can lead to the delivery of local and national policy and strategic targets, as well as clear improvement in health outcomes.

For further information, readers should contact Alison Dale, Clinical and Education Lead, Non-Medical Prescribing and Pharmacy (Alison.Dale@yorksandhumber.nhs.uk)

6:3   A prescribing case history presented during an action learning group

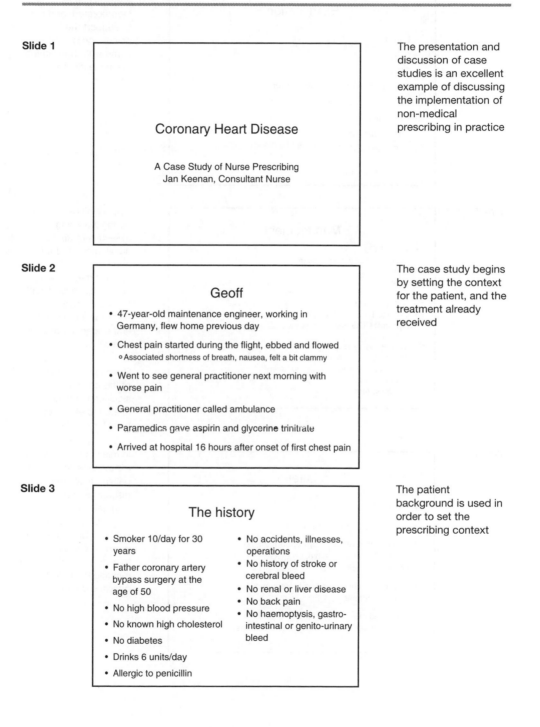

Slide 1

Coronary Heart Disease

A Case Study of Nurse Prescribing
Jan Keenan, Consultant Nurse

The presentation and discussion of case studies is an excellent example of discussing the implementation of non-medical prescribing in practice

Slide 2

Geoff

- 47-year-old maintenance engineer, working in Germany, flew home previous day

- Chest pain started during the flight, ebbed and flowed
  o Associated shortness of breath, nausea, felt a bit clammy

- Went to see general practitioner next morning with worse pain

- General practitioner called ambulance

- Paramedics gave aspirin and glycerine trinitrate

- Arrived at hospital 16 hours after onset of first chest pain

The case study begins by setting the context for the patient, and the treatment already received

Slide 3

The history

- Smoker 10/day for 30 years
- Father coronary artery bypass surgery at the age of 50
- No high blood pressure
- No known high cholesterol
- No diabetes
- Drinks 6 units/day
- Allergic to penicillin

- No accidents, illnesses, operations
- No history of stroke or cerebral bleed
- No renal or liver disease
- No back pain
- No haemoptysis, gastro-intestinal or genito-urinary bleed

The patient background is used in order to set the prescribing context

Slide 4

Examination

- Looks ill
- Grey
- Clammy
- Continued retrosternal discomfort
- BP 125/58 Left; 119/53 Right
- HR 44 bpm, regular
- SaO2 100% on oxygen
- JVP not raised

Clinical examination findings can be incorporated, and tend to support the discussion by immersing the learning set in the clinical situation

Slide 5

Management

- Admit CCU
  - Low molecular weight heparin
  - Aspirin
  - Statin
  - Introduce ACE inhibitor at 24 hours
  - Beta blocker
- Cardiac Troponin I release 14
- Dynamic ECG changes
  - Refer cardiology
  - Load 600 mg Clopidogrel
- Angiography – LAD thrombus, RCA diseased
  - 3 Taxus stents to right coronary artery
  - Discharged
  - Cardiac rehab

Opportunities that arise during a nursing assessment are highlighted, and the need to prescribe specific medication can be discussed, with the lead presenter discussing the need and evidence base for prescribing.

During the discussion of this case study, significant learning related to evidence base for prescribing

Slide 6

Later

- Father died 6 weeks later
- 2 weeks later, more chest pain
- Presented to emergency department, no cardiac Troponin release, no ECG changes – sent home
- Recurrent pain increasing in frequency since Christmas
- Reviewed in nurse-led follow-up clinic within a week of request, with exercise test

---

In relation to the nurse led management of this patient, following discharge from hospital, close follow-up that would not have been available in a medical clinic led to early recognition and management of the patient's deterioration

Slide 7

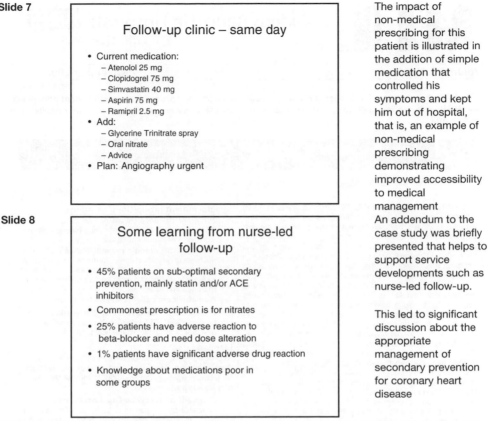

Follow-up clinic – same day

- Current medication:
  - Atenolol 25 mg
  - Clopidogrel 75 mg
  - Simvastatin 40 mg
  - Aspirin 75 mg
  - Ramipril 2.5 mg
- Add:
  - Glycerine Trinitrate spray
  - Oral nitrate
  - Advice
- Plan: Angiography urgent

The impact of non-medical prescribing for this patient is illustrated in the addition of simple medication that controlled his symptoms and kept him out of hospital, that is, an example of non-medical prescribing demonstrating improved accessibility to medical management

Slide 8

Some learning from nurse-led follow-up

- 45% patients on sub-optimal secondary prevention, mainly statin and/or ACE inhibitors
- Commonest prescription is for nitrates
- 25% patients have adverse reaction to beta-blocker and need dose alteration
- 1% patients have significant adverse drug reaction
- Knowledge about medications poor in some groups

An addendum to the case study was briefly presented that helps to support service developments such as nurse-led follow-up.

This led to significant discussion about the appropriate management of secondary prevention for coronary heart disease

6:4 Examples of good practice in keeping prescribers up to date with current evidence and practice

Medicines Information Leaflets provided here as examples are reproduced with kind permission of the authors, Fiona Singleton, Smoking Cessation Advisor, Oxfordshire PCT and Scott Harrison, Lead Pharmacist Anticoagulation, Oxford Radcliffe Hospitals NHS Trust.

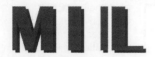

Oxford Radcliffe Hospitals NHS
NHS Trust

Volume 5. No. 5	November 2008

This Medicines Information Leaflet is produced locally to encourage prescribing which is cost effective to the NHS. Information will be given on quality improvement issues and the costs to hospital and community.

Prescribing of Nicotine Replacement Therapy in the Hospital setting

The White Paper 'Smoking Kills' (Department of Health 1998) outlined Government plans to reduce smoking prevalence, with the emphasis being upon cessation support and the part that all health professionals can play. National plans and targets are also reflected in The NHS Plan, Cancer Plan and the National Service Framework for Coronary Heart Disease. Although it is recognised that stopping smoking is the single most effective way to improve health, evidence suggests that patients are not routinely informed of the risk of tobacco use or the potential benefits of quitting. However evidence does suggest that smoking cessation counselling interventions that take place during a period of hospitalisation and that include follow-up support on discharge are effective in helping patients to quit. There-fore, all patients seen either pre-operatively as out-patients or as admissions and in-patients on the ward should all be advised to quit smoking and be offered both support and pharmacotherapy to aid their quit attempt. NICE Guidelines (2008) set out how professionals should support specific groups and people in specific settings, and highlight who should take action. In summary, all patients should be asked about their smoking status, advised to quit and offered Nicotine Replacement Therapy (NRT) if appropriate.

Patients who should receive NRT (inclusion criteria):

Patients who want to quit smoking and require NRT to treat their nicotine dependence.
Trained Smoking Cessation Advisers and Con-sultants can recommend NRT for this purpose.
Patients who are temporarily abstinent - to relieve their withdrawal symptoms to comply with the ORH Smoke Free Policy.
Only Consultants can recommend NRT for this purpose

Patients who should not receive NRT (exclusion criteria):

Patients already using bupropion (Zyban®) or varenicline (Champix®).

Patients with a previous serious reaction to NRT or any of the other ingredients contained in the products, e.g. adhesive in patch

Special patient group/Considerations:

Pregnant patients should not be prescribed the 24-hour patch. During pregnancy patches can be worn for a maximum of 16-hours only.
Patients with chronic generalised skin disease such as psoriasis, chronic dermatitis and urticaria should not be prescribed patches. This also includes patients who have had a previous reaction to transdermal patches.
Non-abstinent patients should discontinue NRT.

Patients with cardiovascular disease should only be prescribed NRT following discussion with a member of the patient's medical team.

Licensed Use
Recent advice from the Committee on Safety of Medi-cines and the Medicines and Healthcare products Regulatory Agency (MHRA 2005), means that NRT may be administered to:

Pregnant or breastfeeding women. Initially, it is advisable for the patient to try to quit without using NRT; if unsuccessful an oral product should be recommended as first-line treatment; however, if the smoker has tried and cannot tolerate an oral product a 16-hour patch can be used.
Patients with a history of diabetes, thyroid disease, cardiovascular disease (initiate under medical supervision), or peptic ulcer disease who are not in the exclusion criteria.

Patients who are aged 12 years or older.

NRT products stocked by Pharmacy:

24-hour Nicotine Patches (NiQuitin CQ®): 21mg, 14mg, 7mg.
16-hour Nicotine Patches (Nicorette®): 15mg, 10mg, 5mg.
Nicotine Lozenges (NiQuitin CQ®) 2mg and 4mg.
Nicotine Inhalator (Nicorette®).

Obtaining NRT in the ORH Trust
NRT will not be dispensed unless a 'Request for Phar-macological Support' form has been completed by a

2

Trained Smoking Cessation Adviser (unless treatment is being initiated by the Consultant, when a Non-Formulary form will need to be completed and telephone advice should be sought from OSAS to clarify what NRT to prescribe.

Tel: 0845 40 80 300 Monday-Friday: 09:00-16:00.

Dose and Frequency

24-hour Nicotine Patch - Apply on waking to dry, non-hairy skin site, removing after 24 hours. Site replacement patch on different area each day. To be used for smokers who would normally have their first cigarette within 30 minutes of waking.

16-hour Nicotine Patch - Apply on waking to dry, non-hairy skin site, removing after 16 hours. Site replacement patch on different area each day. To be used for smokers who would normally have their first cigarette more than 30 minutes after waking and for pregnant smokers.

2mg Nicotine Lozenge – 1 lozenge to be sucked every 1–2 hours, when urge to smoke occurs; maximum of 15 lozenges daily. To be used for smokers who would normally have their first cigarette more than 30 minutes after waking.

4mg Nicotine Lozenge – 1 lozenge to be sucked every 1–2 hours, when urge to smoke occurs; maximum of 15 lozenges daily. To be used for smokers who would normally have their first cigarette within 30 minutes of waking.

Nicotine Inhalator – Each cartridge can be used for approximately 4 sessions, with each cartridge lasting approximately 20 minutes. Maximum usage of 12 cartridges per day

Cautions

Drug Interactions:

Adenosine – NRT may enhance effect.
Cigarette smoking can interact with some medicines, mainly due to polycyclic aromatic hydrocarbons in cigarette smoke that stimulate cytochrome P450 enzymes, and CYP1A2 in particular. A number of medicines are also metabolised by the same isoenzyme, giving a potential interaction when a patient stops or starts smoking.
Most interactions are considered to be of little clinical significance (the MHRA has advised that the inclusion of interaction data is not required in UK prescribing information), but should be borne in mind when someone quits smoking. However some medicines, theophylline and clozapine in particular, may require dosage modification or monitoring when smoking is stopped. Any effect usually happens in weeks 1-4 following cessation of smoking; it is therefore advisable if you are checking bloods for circulating drug concentrations, that you write on the form the date that the patient had their last cigarette.

Benzodiazepines (e.g. chlordiazepoxide, diazepam) – Effect of drug may be enhanced after stopping smoking

Cinacalcet – Inform nephrologists to monitor parathyroid concentrations when stopping smoking

Clozapine – Monitor serum drug concentrations before stopping smoking and 1-2 weeks after. Be alert of in-creased adverse effects and adjust dose accordingly

Insulin – Insulin dose may need to be reduced when stopping smoking.

Opioids – smokers who stop smoking prior to surgery may need increased requirements after surgery.

Theophylline – Stopping smoking may cause an increase in the circulating concentrations of theophylline; therefore, if a patient is taking theophylline their hospital doctor and G.P should be informed that their patient has been supplied with NRT.
Monitor plasma concentrations weekly and adjust dose accordingly until levels are stable when patient stops smoking. It may take several weeks for the enzyme induction to dissipate.

Warfarin – A patient's INR may increase when they stop smoking. Monitor INR more closely.

Chlorpromazine, flecainide, fluvoxamine, haloperidol, olanzapine, quinine, tricyclic antidepressants (e.g clomipramine, imipramine, nortriptylline) smokers may have lower plasma concentrations (increased clearance) so be alert for increased adverse effects when stopping smoking. Reduce dose as necessary if these occur.

Adrenoceptor agonists and antagonists, betablockers, erlotinib, hormonal contraceptives, mexiletine, tamoxifen – No action required

For further Cautions please refer to the BNF. However please note that most Cautions also apply to continuation of cigarette smoking and in all situations the 'risk' of using NRT should be compared to the patient's current risk from smoking.

Side effects of NRT:

The adverse effects of using NRT are usually short term, and may in fact occur as a result of stopping smoking. These could include: nausea, dizziness, headaches, cold and flu like symptoms, dyspepsia and other gastro-intestinal disturbances, hiccups, insomnia, vivid dreams, myalgia, chest pain, blood pressure changes, anxiety and irritability, impaired concentration, dysmenorrhoea.

For references see full Smoking Cessation Guidelines available on the Clinical intranet

Prepared by: Fiona Singleton, Oxfordshire, Smoking Advice Service, T. 0845 40 80 300

With advice from: Danielle Clark, Clinical Effectiveness Pharmacist; Harpreet Rajput, Resident Pharmacist; Vicky Mott, Lead Medicines Information Pharmacist; Jan Keenan, Nurse Consultant Cardiac Medicine, and Marion Elliott, Cardiac Rehabilitation Nurse

Review Date: November 2010

A guide to NRT products and dosages

	Less than 10 cigarettes a day	More than 10 cigarettes a day
Smokes more than 30 mins after waking	VERY LOW DEPENDENCE	LOW DEPENDENCE
Smokes within 30 mins of waking	MEDIUM DEPENDENCE	HIGH DEPENDENCE

DEPENDENCE	PRODUCT	PRESCRIBING INFORMATION (Refer to BNF if use exceeds 6 weeks)
VERY LOW	Inhalator (Nicorette®)	Each cartridge can be used for approximately 4 sessions with each cartridge lasting approximately 20 minutes. Maximum usage of 12 cartridges daily. **PRN medication.**
	2mg Lozenge(NiQuitin CQ®)	1 lozenge to be sucked every 1–2 hours, when urge to smoke occurs; maximum of 15 lozenges daily. **PRN medication.**
LOW	Inhalator (Nicorette®)	Each cartridge can be used for approximately 4 sessions with each cartridge lasting approximately 20 minutes. Maximum usage of 12 cartridges daily. **PRN medication.**
	2mg Lozenge (NiQuitin CQ®)	1 lozenge to be sucked every 1–2 hours, when urge to smoke occurs; maximum of 15 lozenges daily. **PRN medication.**
	16-hour 15mg Patch (Nicor-ette®) for a regular smoker	Apply on waking to dry, non-hairy skin site, removing after 16 hours. Site replacement patch on different area each day. **Regular medication.**
MEDIUM	Inhalator (Nicorette®)	Each cartridge can be used for approximately 4 sessions with each cartridge lasting approximately 20 minutes. Maximum usage of 12 cartridges daily. **PRN medication.**
	4mg Lozenge(NiQuitin CQ®)	1 lozenge to be sucked every 1–2 hours, when urge to smoke occurs; maximum of 15 lozenges daily. **PRN medication.**
	24-hour 14mg Patch (NiQ-uitin CQ®)	Apply on waking to dry, non-hairy skin site, removing after 24 hours. Site replacement patch on different area each day. **Regular medication.**
HIGH	Inhalator (Nicorette®)	Each cartridge can be used for approximately 4 sessions with each cartridge lasting approximately 20 minutes. Maximum usage of 12 cartridges daily. **PRN medication**
	4mg Lozenge (NiQuitin CQ®)	1 lozenge to be sucked every 1–2 hours, when urge to smoke occurs; maximum of 15 lozenges daily. **PRN medication.**
	24-hour 21mg Patch (NiQ-uitin CQ®)	Apply on waking to dry, non-hairy skin site, removing after 24 hours. Site replacement patch on different area each day. **Regular medication.**

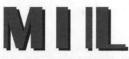 **Oxford Radcliffe Hospitals** *NHS*
NHS Trust

Volume 5. No. 6 (updated)	March 2009

This Medicines Information Leaflet is produced locally to encourage prescribing which is cost effective to the NHS. Information will be given on quality improvement issues and the costs to hospital and community.

Guidelines on when to use and how to monitor Unfractionated Heparin in adults

Heparin remains the most widely used parenteral antithrombotic. The general adoption of low molecular weight (LMWH) represents a significant therapeutic advance in terms of ease and convenience of administration. There may also be some ad-vantages in terms of efficacy and fewer side-effects. This leaflet gives guidance on when to use intravenous unfractionated heparin (UFH) for treatment of thrombosis (it does not address prophylaxis where LMWH is preferred).

Mode of action
Heparin is a glycosaminoglycan, extracted from porcine mucosa and is available as the sodium or calcium salt. Its anticoagulant properties depend on the presence of a specific pentasaccharide sequence which binds with high affinity to antithrombin and potentiates its activity. Metabolism is by a saturable mechanism, involving binding to endothelial cells and clearance by the reticuloendothelial system, and a non-saturable mechanism involving mainly renal clearance. There is no evidence that heparin crosses the placenta.

When to consider using UFH instead of LMWH
LMWHs have replaced UFH as the preferred option in most clinical situations. Use of UFH is only considered in the following situations:
1. Patients who might require their anticoagulation to be stopped rapidly e.g. patients at very high risk of bleeding and those who may require urgent invasive procedures (the half-life of UFH is dose-dependant, around 45-60 min unless renal function is severely impaired).
2. Patients in severe renal failure: titration against the Activated Partial Thromboplastin Time (APTT) is simpler than using LMWH and relying on anti-Xa levels

3. Very obese patients (more than 120kg), in whom dose adjustment of LMWH therapy is less predictable

Indications for intravenous UFH
If patient's condition (see above) warrants the use of UFH rather than LMWH this must be clearly documented in the patient's notes together with the indication for use.

Baseline tests (before treatment)
Measure: APTT; Prothrombin Time (PT); platelet count and potassium.

Dose
Note: Unfractionated heparin dosing is unpredictable and a high percentage of patients will still have APTT results outside the desired range even with careful monitoring. The risks of this must be taken into account when deciding to use UFH rather than LMWH.

Loading dose: 5000 units heparin or 75 units/kg (maximum dose of 10,000 units) Omission of loading dose delays effective anticoagulation.

Maintenance dose: Initially 1400 units heparin per hr or 18 units/kg per hr (maximum dose of 2500 units per hr), equivalent to infusion rate of 1.4mL per hr using infusion solution of 1000 units of heparin per mL.

Cardiology: Reduce initial infusion rate (see below for criteria) to 1000 units per hr (12 units/kg per hr), equivalent to infusion rate of 1mL per hr using infusion solution of 1000 units of heparin per mL :
> Patients receiving aspirin and clopidogrel,
> Patients post-alteplase (rt-PA, tissue-type plasmino-gen activator)
> Patients on heparin during intra aortic balloon pump support
> Patients post abciximab (Reopro®)

2

Note: Patients with prosthetic heart valves requiring heparinisation prior to surgery - discuss initial heparin dose with Cardiologist.

Administration

Loading dose: Give as slow IV bolus over 3-5mins.
Preparation: Use a standardised ready to administer heparin preparation of 1000 units per mL (ie undiluted).

Maintenance dose: Give as continuous IV infusion. Start intravenous infusion at 1400 units per hr =1.4 mL per hr (or 18 units/kg per hr). Adjust dose according to APTT (see monitoring section below and Table 1). A lower initial infusion rate is used for some cardiology patients (see above). The infusion rate must be accurately controlled using a syringe pump.
Preparation:
Use a standardised ready-to-administer heparin preparation of 1000 units per mL. Standard volume of infusion is 25mL (ie 25,000 units in 25mL undiluted). See heparin injectables monograph for complete preparation and administration details.
Once prepared the infusion should only be used for 24 hours and any remaining infusion solution discarded. The infusion must be monitored at hourly intervals using infusion monitoring chart.

Monitoring APTT
The target APTT is 60 – 100´ seconds.
Check APTT 4 hrs after start of infusion, and adjust infusion rate according to **Table 1**.
Recheck APTT 6 hrs after any change of dose (4 hrs if greater than 170 or less than 45) or, if no change required check within 24 h.

Target APTT and infusion rate changes must be documented appropriately. In general ward areas **all dose and infusion rate changes must be hand written on the in-patient drug chart and signed by a doctor.**

Patient Monitoring
Monitor patient for signs of bleeding. Platelet counts should be measured on alternate days from days 4-14 of therapy (see below). Potassium should also be monitored regularly, especially if therapy exceeds 7 days

Table 1: Adjustment of heparin infusion rate based on APTT using infusion solution of 1000 units per mL concentration

APTT (s)	Action
greater than 170	Stop for one hr and reduce infu-sion rate by 300units/hr (0.3 mL/hr)
126-170	Reduce infusion rate by 200 units/hr (0.2 mL/hr)
101-125	Reduce infusion rate by 100 units/hr (0.1 mL/hr)
60-100	No change
45-59	Increase infusion rate by 200 units/hr (0.2 mL/hr)
Less than 45	Give a 500 unit bolus IV and increase infusion rate by 300 units/hr (0.3 mL/hr)

\# *An APTT of 60 – 100 seconds corresponds to 0.35-0.7 anti-Xa units/mL with the current laboratory reagent. It will need to be reviewed when the APTT reagent is changed.*

***Before changing the rate of infusion, check that the initial rate was correct ***

Compatible infusions:
Glucose 5%, Sodium Chloride 0.9%   Heparin is incompatible with a number of medicines including many antibacterials. Contact Medicines Information (Ext 21505) for further advice.

Heparin and intramuscular injections
Intramuscular injections should be avoided in patients receiving anticoagulants, except for adrenaline for severe anaphylaxis.

Contra-Indications
severe liver disease
peptic ulcer
severe / uncontrolled hypertension
known haemorrhagic diathesis
thrombocytopenia
recent cerebral haemorrhage.
injuries to or recent operations to the eyes/ears
central nervous system.
infective endocarditis
active tuberculosis
spinal or epidural anaesthesia

3

Cautions

concomitant medicines that may enhance anticoagulant effect e.g. aspirin, clopidogrel, dipyridamole iloprost, NSAIDs

hepatic impairment

renal impairment

Adverse effects

haemorrhage
thrombocytopenia (see below)
hyperkalaemia (see below)
osteoporosis
alopecia on prolonged use
hypersensitivity reactions (including urticaria, angioedema, and anaphylaxis)

Hyperkalaemia

Inhibition of aldosterone secretion by heparin can result in hyperkalaemia; patients with diabetes mellitus, chronic renal failure, acidosis, raised plasma potassium or those taking potassium-sparing drugs seem to be more susceptible. The risk appears to increase with duration of therapy and the CSM has recommended that the potassium concentration should be measured in patients at risk of hyperkalaemia before starting heparin and monitored regularly thereafter, particularly if heparin is to be continued for longer than 7 days.

Heparin and surgery

In patients with normal renal function intravenous UFH can be stopped 6 hrs before surgery to allow coagulation to return to normal.

Heparin-induced thrombocytopenia(HIT)

Clinically important HIT is immune-mediated and does not usually develop until 5–10 days after starting heparin therapy unless the patient has been exposed to heparin before. HIT can be complicated by thrombosis. All patients who are to receive heparin should have a platelet count on the day of starting treatment. For patients previously exposed to heparin in the last 100 days, obtain a platelet count 24 hrs after starting heparin. For all other patients alternate day platelet counts should be performed from days 4 to 14 of therapy. Signs of HIT include a 50% reduction of platelet count, thrombosis, or skin allergy. If HIT is strongly suspected or confirmed, heparin should be stopped and an alternative anticoagulant should be given. Contact haematology for advice.

Overdose/Reversal

In an emergency the anticoagulant effect of heparin can be inhibited by protamine sulphate. One mg of protamine sulphate inhibits the effect of 100 units of heparin – usually the maximum dose is 50 mg given by slow IV injection (rate not exceeding 5mg per minute)

Switching from UFH to LMWH

If patients are to be switched from intravenous UFH to subcutaneous LMWH, the UFH infusion should be stopped approximately 4 hours before the first dose of LMWH is due (providing patient's renal function is normal and last APTT result is within range i.e. 60-100).

Safe Medication Practice for prescribing Heparin Infusions

Target APTT should be documented
Heparin should always be prescribed with 'UNITS' written in full
Always use standard heparin infusion concentration of 1000 units per 1mL
The prescription must state
✓ Heparin dose in units for bolus dose
✓ Heparin infusion rate in mL per hour
✓ Infusion volume
✓ Route
✓ Time for next APTT
Infusion rate changes must be prescribed by doctor.

Infusion must be changed every 24 hrs

References

Baglin, T., Barrowcliffe, T.W., Cohen, A. & Greaves, M. (2006) Guidelines on the use and monitoring of heparin. Br J Haematol, 133, 19-34.

Sweetman SC (Ed). Martindale: The Complete Drug Reference. 35th Ed, Pharmaceutical Press; London 2007.

Trissel L.A. Handbook on Injectable Drugs. 10th Edition, American Society of Health-System Pharmacists Inc, Bethesda

Prepared by: David Keeling, Consultant Haematologist; Jo Coleman, Medicines Safety Pharmacist; Scott Harrison, Lead Pharmacist - anticoagulation. With advice from: Colin Forfar, Consultant Cardiologist

APPENDIX 7

Keeping Up to Date with Pharmacology

This appendix contains a list of useful websites that support continuing professional development in relation to prescribing practice, as well as the answers to the pharmacology self-test, presented in Chapter 7.

7:1   Useful websites

Bandolier
  http://www.library.nhs.uk
BMJ Best Treatments
  http://www.besttreatments.bmj.com
BMJ Clinical Evidence
  http://www.clinicalevidence.bmj.com
BNF
  http://www.bnf.org
Cochrane Library
  http://www.cochrane.org
Dr Companion
  http://www.dr.companion.com
Drug & Therapeutics Bulletin
  http://www.dtb.bmj.com
InfoPOEMS & InfoRetriever
  http://www.infopoems.com
MeRec
  http://www.npc.co.uk/merec.htm
National Institute for Clinical Excellence (NICE)
  http://www.nice.org.uk

National Prescribing Centre (NPC)
  http://www.npc.co.uk

National Prescribing Interactive Site
  http://www.npci.org.uk

NHS National Electronic Library for Health
  http://www.library.nhs.uk

Clinical Knowledge Summaries
  http://www.prodigy.nhs.uk

7:2   Answers to pharmacology self-test multi-choice questions

1. True	**14.** a
2. b	**15.** a
3. b	**16.** b
4. d	**17.** d
5. a	**18.** a
6. c	**19.** c
7. b	**20.** b
8. a	**21.** b
9. d	**22.** b
10. c	**23.** a
11. c	**24.** d
12. c	**25.** c
13. a	

7:3   Acknowledgements

We are grateful to Akin Adeniaran, Pharmacist and Senior Lecturer, Oxford Brookes University, for developing this example of pharmacology self-test.

APPENDIX 8

Organising CPD for Non-Medical Prescribers in a General Practice Setting

In Chapter 8, Mandy Fry discusses several approaches to keeping up to date with prescribing practice in a community and general practice setting. In this appendix, with the kind permission of the authors, we include two particularly good examples of prescribing newsletters that are currently in Primary Care Trust (PCT) circulation. These are of interest for two reasons – firstly, as an example of good practice in communication, and secondly, from the perspective of clinical interest in areas of prescribing that will relate to the practice of many readers.

8:1 Prescribing points

Two examples of communication of prescribing issues in a primary care setting. We are very grateful to Sarah Wilds, Primary Care Prescribing Lead, Oxfordshire PCT, to Jane Bennett and Sian Hills, and to the Medicines Management Team of Oxfordshire PCT for their permission to reproduce current issues of 'Prescribing Points'.

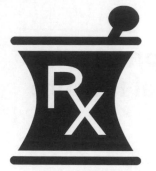

Prescribing Points

A NEWSLETTER FOR ALL HEALTH CARE PROFESSIONALS IN OXFORDSHIRE, WRITTEN BY THE MEDICINES MANAGEMENT TEAM, OXFORDSHIRE PCT, JUBILEE HOUSE, OXFORD BUSINESS PARK SOUTH, OXFORD, OX4 2LH.

MAY 2008	**VOLUME 17.09** Written by Jane Bennett & Sara Wilds Therapeutics Team
In this issue:	**British Guidelines on the Management of Asthma**
Page 1	Background
Page 2 - 6	The Pharmacological Management of Asthma
Page 6	Inhaler devices
Page 7	Summary of Stepwise Management of Asthma in **Adults**
Page 8	Summary of Stepwise Management of Asthma in **children (5-12 years)**
Page 9	Summary of Stepwise Management of Asthma in **children (0-5 years)**

Background

The British Thoracic Society and the Scottish Intercollegiate Guidelines Network have jointly published a new British Guideline on the Management of Asthma.[1i] This replaces the previous 2003 version which was published as a supplement to Thorax,[2] and the subsequent on-line versions, the last of which was written in July 2007 [3]. The guidelines are divided into ten sections. The sections which include changes from the last version are *indicated in italics*

> *diagnosis and monitoring,*
> *non-pharmacological management,*
> *pharmacological management,*
> **inhaler devices**
> **management of acute asthma**
> **special situations incl.** *difficult asthma,* **asthma in pregnancy, labour and breastfeeding and occupational asthma**
> *organisation and delivery of care, and audit,*
> *patient education and self-management*
> **development of the guidelines**

We have restricted discussions in this newsletter to the pharmacological management of asthma **and** inhaler devices **(excluding the management of acute asthma) but the full guideline and a quick reference guide can be downloaded from www.brit-thoracic.org.uk or www.sign.ac.uk .**

[1] British Thoracic Society and Scottish Intercollegiate Guidelines Network. British Guideline on the Management of Asthma. Thorax 2008; 63 (Suppl 4): iv1-iv121. Also available via www.brit-thoracic.org.uk/Portals/0/Clinical%20Information/Asthma/Guidelines/asthma_final2008.pdf and www.sign.ac.uk/pdf/sign101.pdf.

[2] British Thoracic Society and Scottish Intercollegiate Guidelines Network. British Guideline on the Management of Asthma. Thorax 2003; 58 (Suppl 1): i1-i94.

[3] **British Thoracic Society and Scottish Intercollegiate Guidelines Network. British Guideline on the Management of Asthma. Revised edition July 2007. Accessed via** www.brit-thoracic.org.uk/Portals/0/Clinical%20Information/Asthma/Guidelines/asthma_fullguideline2007.pdf

The Pharmacological Management of Asthma

Significant changes to this section of the guideline were published on-line in July 2007 and the new 2008 version includes only a small number of additional revisions. The major changes made in 2007 and 2008 are *highlighted in italics*.

The aim of asthma management is control of the disease newly defined as:

> *no daytime symptoms,*
> *no night time awakening due to asthma,*
> *no need for rescue medication,*
> *no exacerbations,*
> *no limitations on activity*
> *normal lung function*
> *with minimal side effects*

Patients should start treatment at the step most appropriate to the initial severity of their asthma. The aim is to achieve early control and to maintain control by stepping up treatment as necessary and stepping down when control is good.

All doses of inhaled steroids refer to **beclometasone (BDP)** given via **CFC-MDIs (metered dose inhalers)**. Although now almost phased out, this is the device used in most of the evidence base that supports current asthma management. **Adjustment to dose will have to be made for other corticosteroids and other devices.**

STEP 1: MILD INTERMITTENT ASTHMA

Prescribe an inhaled short-acting β_2 agonist as short term reliever therapy for all patients with symptomatic asthma
As required is at least as good as regular administration
Patients with high usage of inhaled short-acting β_2 agonists should have their asthma management reviewed
Using two or more canisters of β_2 agonists per month or >10-12 puffs per day is a marker of poorly controlled asthma

STEP 2: INTRODUCTION OF REGULAR PREVENTER THERAPY

Inhaled steroids

Inhaled steroids are the recommended preventer drug for adults and children for achieving overall treatment goals.

Many children with recurrent episodes of viral induced wheezing in infancy do not go on to have chronic atopic asthma. The majority do not require treatment with regular inhaled steroids.

Inhaled steroids should be considered for adults and children aged 5-12 and children under the age of 5 with any of the following features:

> Using inhaled short-acting β_2 agonists three times a week or more
> Symptomatic three times a week or more
> Waking one night a week
> Exacerbation of asthma requiring oral corticosteroids in the last two years (adults and children 5-12 years only)

Patients should be started at a dose of inhaled steroids appropriate to the severity of disease.

A reasonable starting dose will be usually 400mcg BDP per day for adults and 200mcg for children. In children under five years, higher doses may be required if there are problems in obtaining consistent drug delivery.

The dose should be titrated to the lowest dose at which effective asthma control is maintained.

Most inhaled steroids should be given twice daily although a once daily regime can be used (using the same total daily dose) if good control is established.

Safety of inhaled steroids

The safety of inhaled steroids is of crucial importance and a balance between benefits and risks for each individual needs to be assessed. Account should be taken of other topical steroid therapy.

Adults: there is little evidence that doses below 800mcg BDP per day cause any short-term detrimental effects apart from the local side-effects. The possibility of long-term effects on the bone has been raised but has not been proven. The dose of inhaled steroid should be titrated to the lowest dose at which effective control of asthma is maintained.

Children: administration of inhaled steroids at or above 400mcg BDP a day may be associated with systemic side-effects. These may include growth failure and adrenal suppression. Clinical adrenal insufficiency has been identified in a small number of children who became acutely unwell at the time of intercurrent illness. Most had been treated with high doses of inhaled corticosteroid. The dose or duration of inhaled corticosteroid that places a child at risk of clinical adrenal insufficiency is unknown. But it is likely to occur at ≥800mcg BDP / day. At higher doses, add-on agents, eg. long-acting β2-agonists should be considered.

> Monitor height of children on high doses of steroid on a regular basis
> The lowest dose of inhaled steroid compatible with maintaining disease control should be used.

When treating children with 800microgram or more per day of BDP or equivalent (rather than 1,000microgram as in the previous version of the guideline) the guideline advises that:

- Specific written advice about steroid replacement in the event of a severe intercurrent illness should be part of the management plan.
- The child should be under the care of a specialist paediatrician for the duration of the treatment.

Comparison of inhaled steroids

Betamethasone and budesonide are approximately equivalent in clinical practice, although there may be a variation in delivery devices, and a ratio of 1:1 should assumed when switching between the two.

Fluticasone provides equal clinical activity to BDP at half the dosage. The evidence that it causes fewer side-effects at doses with equal clinical effect is limited.

Mometasone is a new inhaled steroid that appears to provide equal clinical activity to BDP at half the dosage. The relative safety of mometasone has not been fully established.

Ciclesonide is a new inhaled steroid. Evidence from clinical trials suggests that it has less systemic activity and fewer local oropharyngeal side-effects than conventional inhaled steroids. The clinical benefit of this is not clear as the exact efficacy to safety ratio compared to other inhaled steroids has not been fully established.

Non-CFC BDP is available in more than one preparation and the potency relative to CFC BDP is not consistent.

Smoking

Clinicians should be aware that higher doses of inhaled steroids may be needed in patients who are smokers or ex-smokers

Inhaled corticosteroids are first choice preventer drug. Long acting β_2-agonist (LABA) should not be used without inhaled corticosteroids.

STEP 3: INITIAL ADD-ON THERAPY

Before initiating a new drug therapy practitioners should recheck compliance, inhaler technique and eliminate trigger factors.

Criteria for introduction of add-on therapy

No exact dose of inhaled steroid can be deemed the correct dose at which to add another therapy. Many patients will benefit more from add-on therapy than from increasing inhaled steroids above doses as low as 200mcg per day. At doses of inhaled steroid above 800mcg per day side effects become more frequent.

Add-on therapy

The first choice as add-on therapy to inhaled steroids in adults and children (5-12years) is an inhaled long-acting β_2-agonist (LABA) which should be considered before going above a dose of 400mcg BDP per day and certainly before going above 800mcg BDP per day.

For children under 5 years taking inhaled steroids 200-400mcg BDP per day consider addition of a leukotriene receptor antagonist.

In children under 2 consider proceeding to step 4.

An inhaled long-acting β_2-agonist should only be started in patients who are already on an inhaled corticosteroid.

- If there is no response, the LABA should be stopped and the dose of inhaled steroid increased to 800mcg BDP per day in adults (400mcg per day in children) if not already on this dose.

- If there is a response to the LABA but control still remains suboptimal, continue with LABA and increase the dose of the inhaled steroid to 800mcg BDP per day (adults) and 400mcg BDP per day (children 5-12 years) if not already on these doses

- If control still remains inadequate after stopping a LABA and increasing the dose of inhaled steroid, consider sequential trials of add-on therapy, ie leukotriene receptor antagonists, theophyllines or slow-release β_2 agonist tablets (adults only)

Combination inhalers

There is no difference in efficacy in giving inhaled steroid and a LABA in combination or in separate inhalers.

Combination inhalers containing a steroid and long-acting β-2 agonist are useful in ensuring that beta-2 agonists are not used without concomitant inhaled steroid.

In adult patients at step 3 who are poorly controlled, the use of budesonide/ formoterol in a single inhaler as rescue medication instead of a short-acting beta2 agonist, in addition to its regular use as a controller treatment, is an effective treatment option. This management technique has not been investigated with other combination inhalers. Before instituting this management careful patient education is required.

(It is important to note that the guidance says this is an **option** for **patients at step 3** who are **poorly controlled.** This refers to patients who have already moved from step 2 to step 3 (ie they have previously needed to move from regular inhaled steroid alone to regular inhaled steroid plus regular long-acting beta2 agonist [LABA]), and whose asthma is uncontrolled with this regime, as an alternative to moving to step 4. Note also that not all patients respond to LABAs, in which case an alternative approach is required - see the guideline).

STEP 4: POOR CONTROL ON MODERATE DOSE OF INHALED STEROID + ADD ON THERAPY: ADDITION OF A FOURTH DRUG

If control remains inadequate on a combination of a short-acting $\beta2$ agonist, 800mcg BDP daily (adults) and 400mcg BDP daily (children) of an inhaled steroid plus an additional drug (usually a LABA), the following interventions should be considered for adults and children (5-12 years):

- Increasing inhaled steroids to 2000mcg BDP per day (adults) or 800mcg (children 5 – 12 years). At high doses of inhaled steroid via an MDI, a spacer should be used.
- Leukotriene receptor antagonists
- Theophyllines
- Slow-release $\beta2$ agonist tablets (caution if on long-acting $\beta2$ agonist)

If a trial of an add-on treatment is ineffective, stop the drug (or in the case of the inhaled steroid, reduce to the original dose)

Before proceeding to step 5, consider referring patients with inadequately controlled asthma, especially children, to specialist care.

STEP 5: CONTINUOUS OR FREQUENT USE OF ORAL STEROIDS

For the small number of patients not controlled at step 4, use daily steroid tablets in the lowest dose providing adequate control.

Patients on long-term steroid tablets (ie > 3 months) or requiring frequent courses (ie 3 or 4 per year) will be at risk of systemic side-effects.

- Blood pressure should be monitored
- Diabetes mellitus and hyperlipidaemia may occur
- Bone mineral density should be monitored (when a significant reduction occurs, treatment with a bisphosphonate should be initiated)
- Growth should be monitored in children
- Cataracts should be screened for (in adults and in children)

Steroid tablet-sparing medication

In adults, the recommended method of eliminating or reducing the dose of steroid tablets is inhaled steroids, at doses up to 2000mcg BDP if required.

In children aged 5-12 years, careful consideration should be given before going above doses of 800mcg inhaled BDP per day.

There is a role for a trial of treatment with:

- LABA plus
- Leukotriene receptor antagonists plus
- theophyllines

for six weeks. They should be stopped if no improvement in steroid dose, symptoms or lung function is detected.

Other treatments such as methotrexate, ciclosporin, oral gold, decrease long-term steroid tablet requirements but they all have significant side-effects and no persisting benefit has been seen after stopping them.

Anti-TNF alpha therapy has been investigated in severe asthma but these studies are too small and too short term to allow recommendation of anti-TNF therapy outside the context of a controlled clinical trial.

Steroid formulations
Prednisolone is the most widely used steroid tablets used for maintenance therapy in chronic asthma. There is no evidence that alternate day dosing produces fewer side-effects than once daily dosing.

STEPPING DOWN

Stepping down therapy once asthma is controlled is recommended, but often not implemented leaving some patients overtreated

Regular review of patients as treatment is stepped down is important. When deciding which drug to step down first and at what rate the severity of asthma, side-effects of treatment, time on treatment, beneficial effect achieved and patient preference should all be taken into account.

Patients should be maintained at the lowest possible dose of inhaled steroid.

Reduction in inhaled steroid dose should be slow as patients deteriorate at different rates. Reductions should be considered every 3 months, decreasing the dose by approximately 25-50% each time

---

Inhaler Devices

Prescribe inhalers only after patients have received training in the use of the device and have demonstrated satisfactory technique

β_2 AGONIST DELIVERY

Acute Asthma
Children and adults with mild and moderate exacerbations of asthma should be treated by pMDI + spacer with doses titrated according to clinical response

Stable Asthma
- For children aged 0-5, there is no evidence, comparing nebulisers and other inhaler devices, sufficiently robust to draw any conclusions for pMDI vs DPI (dry powder inhaler).
- In children aged 5-12, pMDI + spacer is as effective as any other hand held inhaler.
- In adults, pMDI ± spacer is as effective as any other hand held inhaler, but patients may prefer some types of DPI.

INHALED STEROID DELIVERY

- Although there is no comparative data on inhaled steroids for stable asthma in children under 5 years, pMDI + spacer are the preferred method of delivery of β_2 agonists or inhaled steroids. A face mask is required until the child can breath reproducibly using the spacer mouthpiece. Where this is ineffective, a nebuliser may be required.

- In children aged 5-12 years, pMDI + spacer is as effective as any DPI.

- In adults, a pMDI ± spacer is as effective as any DPI.

USE AND CARE OF SPACERS

Spacers should be cleaned monthly rather than weekly or performance is adversely affected. They should be washed in detergent and allowed to dry in air. The mouthpiece should be wiped clean of detergent before use.

Spacers should be replaced at least every 12 months but some may be need changing at 6 months

Management of Asthma in Adults

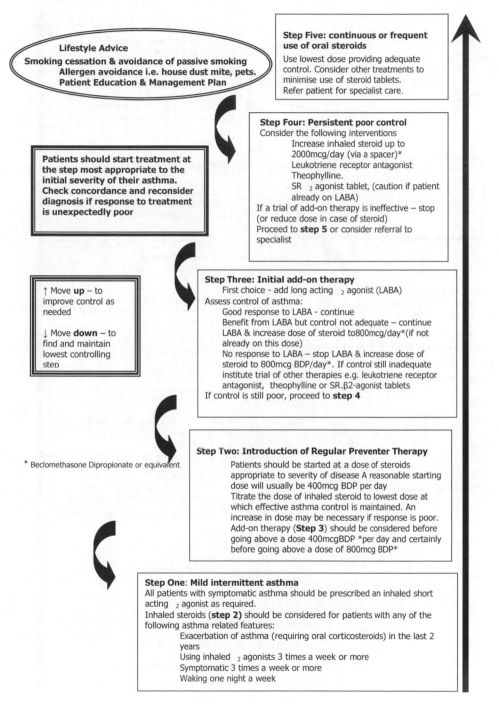

Step Five: continuous or frequent use of oral steroids
Use lowest dose providing adequate control. Consider other treatments to minimise use of steroid tablets.
Refer patient for specialist care.

Lifestyle Advice
Smoking cessation & avoidance of passive smoking
Allergen avoidance i.e. house dust mite, pets.
Patient Education & Management Plan

Patients should start treatment at the step most appropriate to the initial severity of their asthma. Check concordance and reconsider diagnosis if response to treatment is unexpectedly poor

Step Four: Persistent poor control
Consider the following interventions
Increase inhaled steroid up to 2000mcg/day (via a spacer)*
Leukotriene receptor antagonist
Theophylline.
SR ₂ agonist tablet, (caution if patient already on LABA)
If a trial of add-on therapy is ineffective – stop (or reduce dose in case of steroid)
Proceed to **step 5** or consider referral to specialist

↑ Move **up** – to improve control as needed

↓ Move **down** – to find and maintain lowest controlling step

Step Three: Initial add-on therapy
First choice - add long acting ₂ agonist (LABA)
Assess control of asthma:
Good response to LABA - continue
Benefit from LABA but control not adequate – continue LABA & increase dose of steroid to800mcg/day*(if not already on this dose)
No response to LABA – stop LABA & increase dose of steroid to 800mcg BDP/day*. If control still inadequate institute trial of other therapies e.g. leukotriene receptor antagonist, theophylline or SR.β2-agonist tablets
If control is still poor, proceed to **step 4**

* Beclomethasone Dipropionate or equivalent

Step Two: Introduction of Regular Preventer Therapy
Patients should be started at a dose of steroids appropriate to severity of disease A reasonable starting dose will usually be 400mcg BDP per day
Titrate the dose of inhaled steroid to lowest dose at which effective asthma control is maintained. An increase in dose may be necessary if response is poor.
Add-on therapy (**Step 3**) should be considered before going above a dose 400mcgBDP *per day and certainly before going above a dose of 800mcg BDP*

Step One: Mild intermittent asthma
All patients with symptomatic asthma should be prescribed an inhaled short acting ₂ agonist as required.
Inhaled steroids (**step 2**) should be considered for patients with any of the following asthma related features:
Exacerbation of asthma (requiring oral corticosteroids) in the last 2 years
Using inhaled ₂ agonists 3 times a week or more
Symptomatic 3 times a week or more
Waking one night a week

Management of Asthma in Children Aged 5 -12 years

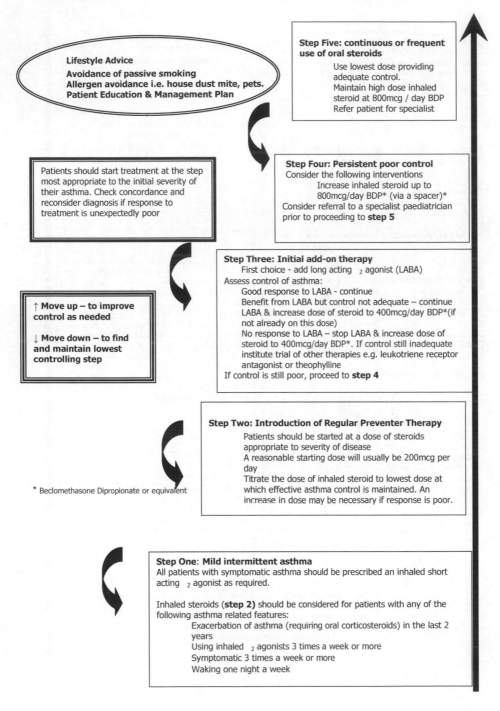

Lifestyle Advice
Avoidance of passive smoking
Allergen avoidance i.e. house dust mite, pets.
Patient Education & Management Plan

Step Five: continuous or frequent use of oral steroids
Use lowest dose providing adequate control.
Maintain high dose inhaled steroid at 800mcg / day BDP
Refer patient for specialist

Patients should start treatment at the step most appropriate to the initial severity of their asthma. Check concordance and reconsider diagnosis if response to treatment is unexpectedly poor

Step Four: Persistent poor control
Consider the following interventions
Increase inhaled steroid up to 800mcg/day BDP* (via a spacer)*
Consider referral to a specialist paediatrician prior to proceeding to **step 5**

Step Three: Initial add-on therapy
First choice - add long acting $_2$ agonist (LABA)
Assess control of asthma:
Good response to LABA - continue
Benefit from LABA but control not adequate – continue LABA & increase dose of steroid to 400mcg/day BDP*(if not already on this dose)
No response to LABA – stop LABA & increase dose of steroid to 400mcg/day BDP*. If control still inadequate institute trial of other therapies e.g. leukotriene receptor antagonist or theophylline
If control is still poor, proceed to **step 4**

↑ **Move up – to improve control as needed**

↓ **Move down – to find and maintain lowest controlling step**

Step Two: Introduction of Regular Preventer Therapy
Patients should be started at a dose of steroids appropriate to severity of disease
A reasonable starting dose will usually be 200mcg per day
Titrate the dose of inhaled steroid to lowest dose at which effective asthma control is maintained. An increase in dose may be necessary if response is poor.

* Beclomethasone Dipropionate or equivalent

Step One: Mild intermittent asthma
All patients with symptomatic asthma should be prescribed an inhaled short acting $_2$ agonist as required.

Inhaled steroids (**step 2)** should be considered for patients with any of the following asthma related features:
Exacerbation of asthma (requiring oral corticosteroids) in the last 2 years
Using inhaled $_2$ agonists 3 times a week or more
Symptomatic 3 times a week or more
Waking one night a week

Management of Asthma in Children under 5 years

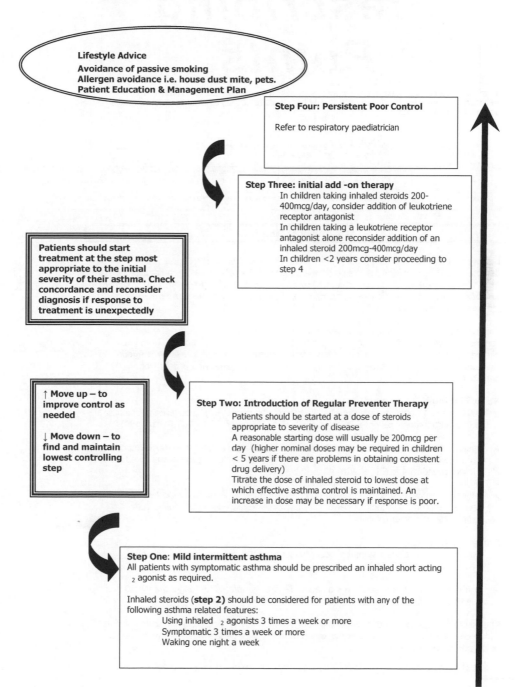

Lifestyle Advice
Avoidance of passive smoking
Allergen avoidance i.e. house dust mite, pets.
Patient Education & Management Plan

Step Four: Persistent Poor Control

Refer to respiratory paediatrician

Step Three: initial add -on therapy
In children taking inhaled steroids 200-
400mcg/day, consider addition of leukotriene
receptor antagonist
In children taking a leukotriene receptor
antagonist alone reconsider addition of an
inhaled steroid 200mcg-400mcg/day
In children <2 years consider proceeding to
step 4

**Patients should start
treatment at the step most
appropriate to the initial
severity of their asthma. Check
concordance and reconsider
diagnosis if response to
treatment is unexpectedly**

↑ **Move up – to
improve control as
needed**

↓ **Move down – to
find and maintain
lowest controlling
step**

Step Two: Introduction of Regular Preventer Therapy
Patients should be started at a dose of steroids
appropriate to severity of disease
A reasonable starting dose will usually be 200mcg per
day (higher nominal doses may be required in children
< 5 years if there are problems in obtaining consistent
drug delivery)
Titrate the dose of inhaled steroid to lowest dose at
which effective asthma control is maintained. An
increase in dose may be necessary if response is poor.

Step One: Mild intermittent asthma
All patients with symptomatic asthma should be prescribed an inhaled short acting
₂ agonist as required.

Inhaled steroids (**step 2**) should be considered for patients with any of the
following asthma related features:
Using inhaled   ₂ agonists 3 times a week or more
Symptomatic 3 times a week or more
Waking one night a week

Prescribing
Points

A NEWSLETTER FOR ALL HEALTH CARE PROFESSIONALS IN OXFORDSHIRE, WRITTEN BY THE MEDICINES MANAGEMENT TEAM, OXFORDSHIRE PCT, JUBILEE HOUSE, OXFORD BUSINESS PARK SOUTH, OXFORD, OX4 2LH.

MARCH 2008	VOLUME 17.06 Written by Sian Hills Therapeutics Team
In this issue:	**Recent Antimicrobial Prescribing Issues**
Pages 1 and 2	Treatment of Sinusitis
Page 3	Medicines Management Team Monitoring of Primary Care Prescribing of Out of Formulary Antibiotics
Page 3	Draft NICE Guideline on the prescribing of antibiotics for self-limiting respiratory tract infections in adults and children in primary care
Page 4	Current local guidance on the prescribing of antibiotics for self-limiting respiratory tract infections in adults and children in primary care

Treatment of Sinusitis

Last week, the national media reported on an analysis published in The Lancet which demonstrated that antibiotics make no difference even if the patient has been ill for more than seven days. Headlines appeared including: `Sinus bug antibiotics no good` 'and 'Doctors *should cut down on antibiotic prescriptions for Sinusitis because the antibiotics do not work, researchers say.*'

This Lancet meta-analysis of nine published trials suggests that primary-care physicians continue to over prescribe antibiotics for acute sinusitis because distinction between viral and bacterial sinus infection is difficult. The study was undertaken to assess whether common signs and symptoms can be used to identify a subgroup of patients who benefit from antibiotics.

Study Findings

> **NNT is 15:** 15 patients with sinusitis-like complaints would have to be given antibiotics before an additional patient was cured (95% CI NNT [benefit] 7 to NNT [harm] 190).

> Patients with purulent discharge in the pharynx took longer to cure than those without this sign; the NNT was 8 patients with this sign before one additional patient was cured (95% CI NNT [benefit] 4 to NNT [harm] 47).

> Patients who were older, reported symptoms for longer, or those that reported more severe symptoms also took longer to cure but were no more likely to benefit from antibiotics than other patients.

Study Interpretation

> Common clinical signs & symptoms cannot identify patients with sinusitis for whom treatment is clearly justified.

> Antibiotics are not justified even if a patient reports symptoms for longer than 7–10 days due to side effects, costs and the risk of resistance.

The media reports suggest that sinusitis is very common - often occurring after colds or flu with 1-5% of adults diagnosed every year and round 90% of people with sinusitis in the UK being prescribed antibiotics.

Study leader, Dr Jim Young said: "If a patient comes to the GP and says they have had the complaint for seven to 10 days that's not a good enough reason for giving them the antibiotic." He added *it would be reasonable for GPs to advise patients to come back if symptoms got worse or went on for another week.*

Co-author, Dr Ian Williamson, a GP in Southampton and researcher at Southampton University, said sinusitis is a horrible condition with people expected to get antibiotics from their GP to help them but that "Antibiotics really don't look as if they work. and that although we have found that antibiotics aren't effective for sore throats and ear infections that sinusitis, which is similar, is the one condition that people are slightly more die hard about."

Antibiotics and nasal steroids of little/no benefit for acute sinusitis (Williamson IG, Rumsby K, Benge S, et al. Antibiotics and topical nasal steroid for treatment of acute maxillary sinusitis. An RCT: JAMA 2007;298(21):2487-2496.)

Clinical Question: Are antibiotics or nasal steroids truly beneficial in the treatment of acute maxillary sinusitis?

Key Details:

➢ Currently published studies evaluating drug therapy for acute maxillary sinusitis have been conducted in secondary settings with x-ray confirmed cases, and thus may not be generalisable to the primary care setting.

➢ This study enrolled patients older than 15 years meeting clinical criteria for uncomplicated acute maxillary sinusitis. Diagnostic criteria from a previously validated predictive tool include the presence or absence of purulent nasal discharge with unilateral predominance, local pain with unilateral predominance, purulent bilateral nasal discharge, and pus on inspection of the nose.

➢ Patients (n = 240) meeting a minimum of 2 positive criteria randomly received (concealed allocation assignment) either antibiotics (amoxicillin 500 mg 3 times daily for 7 days) and nasal steroids (budesonide 200 mug in each nostril once daily for 10 days), active antibiotic and placebo nasal steroid, placebo antibiotic and active nasal steroid, or placebo antibiotic and placebo nasal steroid. Patients masked to treatment group assignment self-reported outcomes using a daily diary. Complete follow-up occurred for 86% of patients at 6 weeks.

➢ Using intention-to-treat analysis, at 10 days there *were no significant differences reported between any of the groups for 11 symptom variables*, including nasal blockage, discharge, unpleasant taste/smell, pain, quality of life, or headache. The time to overall cure with no symptoms for all 11 items was also similar in all 4 groups. The study was 80% powered to detect a small clinical effect on a total symptom scale.

Bottom Line:

➢ In this government funded double blinded, allocation concealed RCT study conducted in the out-patient setting, the largest published non-pharmaceutically funded randomised controlled trial, *antibiotics and nasal steroids were equal to placebo treatment for acute maxillary sinusitis in adults and adolescents, 15 years and older*.

➢ In clinical practice it is often difficult to convince patients that only the "tincture of time" is needed to treat their sinus infection. However, in this era of publicly exposed concerns about increasing antibiotic resistance and "super bugs," taking a few extra moments for explanation and empathy may reassure many patients that antibiotics and nasal steroids are unnecessary. (LOE = 1b)

Although it is well acknowledged that prescribers had been working hard to reduce antibiotic use for sinusitis in recent years it is also accepted that there are probably still too many antibiotics prescribed and that these studies may give reassurance to prescribers that even if patients have specific symptoms, it's unlikely antibiotics are going to make a dramatic difference."

Oxfordshire PCT Current Local Guidance on the Treatment of Sinusitis

Oxfordshire PCT guidance suggests that:
- Viruses account for over 50% of these infections
- Symptomatic benefit of antibiotics is small and that 69% of cases resolve without antibiotics; and 84% resolve with antibiotics.[A+]
- Antibiotics should be reserved for severe[B+] cases or symptoms longer than 10 days.
- **Cochrane review concludes that amoxicillin and phenoxymethylpenicillin have similar efficacy to other recommended antibiotics.**
- 1st line therapy is suggested as amoxicillin 500mg tds for 7 days, with 2nd line therapy suggested as erythromycin (if allergic to penicillin) 500mg BD (or 250mg QDS) or oxytetracycline (not for children or in pregnancy) 250mg QDS for 7 days

The National Institute for Clinical and health Excellence (NICE) published draft guidance this week advising GPs not to prescribe antibiotics but to consider in some circumstances the issuing of delayed prescriptions which patients can use if they do not get better.

Primary Care Prescribing of Out of Formulary Antibiotics

A recent review by the DoH HCAI Team of PCT activity related to Healthcare Associated Infections from both a provider and commissioner perspective has identified a number of areas of challenge which require PCT focus to improve. This includes an area related to prescribing:

The DH HCAI Team noted significant challenges related to the effective control of high risk antibiotics within the provider care services and that the PCT should consider more stringent monitoring of high risk and out of formulary antibiotics.

As a result, with regard to primary care prescribing, monthly reviews of NHS Business Services Authority Antibiotic Prescribing will be carried out by the Medicines Management Team and discussions put in place to ascertain the rationale for certain out of formulary antibiotic prescribing.

(Other measures are also currently being considered and implemented with regard to community hospital and acute trust prescribing of high risk / out of formulary antibiotics)

From recent review of December 2007 prescribing data it was ascertained that *molifloxacin was prescribed by a number of practices within Oxfordshire PCT* (Ten prescriptions issued by four practices at a total cost of £300.).

Molifloxacin is not included within the revised antimicrobial guidelines and as with all quinolones associated with increased incidence of CDAD and MRSA.

The BNF suggests that molifolxacin should be used for treating acute exacerbations of chronic bronchitis only if conventional treatment has failed or is contra-indicated and for 2nd line treatment of community acquired pneumonia.

Local guidance suggests that for both community acquired pneumonia and acute exacerbations of chronic bronchitis, amoxicillin should be considered 1st line, erythromycin or oxytetracycline 2nd line and clarithromycin 3rd line

---

Practice consideration for practices currently prescribing molifloxacin: Review *prescribing to ensure that prescribing follows local guidance or that exceptions for prescribing out of line with local guidance are clearly documented on the patients' clinical record.*

**Draft NICE Guideline on the prescribing of antibiotics
for self-limiting respiratory tract infections in adults and children in primary care**

NICE has recently issued a draft clinical practice guideline on the prescribing of antibiotics for self-limiting respiratory tract infections in adults and children in primary care for consultation; comments from registered stakeholders are invited up until 8th April 2008.

The use of three antibiotic management strategies is discussed:
➢ No prescribing,
➢ Delayed prescribing
➢ Immediate prescribing.

It suggests that a **no antibiotic** or **a delayed antibiotic prescribing strategy** should be negotiated for patients with the following conditions:
• Acute otitis media
• Acute cough/acute bronchitis
• Acute sore throat
• Acute sinusitis
• Common cold

The guidance also discusses situations in which immediate prescribing is appropriate (e.g. systemically unwell, high risk of serious complications, aged above 65 years with two or more risk factors).

Current local Oxfordshire guidance would appear to be consistent with this draft NICE Guideline however it will be necessary to review local guidance once this draft NICE clinical guideline is finalised.

Practice Consideration: Is prescribing of antibiotics for the management of self-limiting respiratory tract infections in adults and children within the practice by all prescribers and clinicians and non clinical staff that influence the prescribing process consistent with the draft NICE Guideline?

A Reminder of Local Guidance:
*See Prescribing Points Volume 16.21 December 2007 Common Primary Care
Respiratory Infections: General Principles to consider before prescribing antibiotics*

➢ Prescribing for **respiratory tract infections accounts for a high proportion of antibiotic** use in the UK.
➢ Many of these conditions are highly likely **to be due to viral infection or be self-limiting conditions with a low absolute risk of complications.**
➢ Prescribing antibiotics widely in these cases **increases resistance** (a major threat to public health)
➢ Prescribing antibiotics widely **puts patients at risk of adverse reactions** from the treatment that may be worse than the infection itself!

> On average 1 patient in 17 prescribed an antibiotic suffers a significant adverse effect.
> **Often the greatest problem for healthcare professionals is working out which infections are most likely to be bacterial or who may develop a complication.**

The previous December 2007 'Prescribing Points' newsletter (Vol 16.21) aims to outline some simple, well accepted techniques to assist working out which infections are most likely to be bacterial or who may develop a complication, whilst supporting a decreased use of antibiotics in conditions where they are often not required.

Maintain clear objectives when prescribing antibiotics:
> Use to treat / prevent *serious illness* and ensure a lower threshold for prescribing when considering high risk groups such as the elderly, very young and respiratory / cardiac patients.
> Use to *reduce suffering* in a patient presenting with *severe symptoms*: *consider* prescribing for *severe* sore throats, *severe* ear infections.
> Use to *prevent complications* of infections.

Prescribe rationally:
> If *confident an antibiotic will help achieve any of the above objectives, then prescribe*.
> If *unsure whether or not antibiotics will help*, then *issue a deferred prescription*.
> If *sure antibiotics will not help*, then *do not* prescribe.
> Use *first line antibiotics listed in the 'Oxfordshire Prescribing Guidelines* for *the use of Antimicrobial Agents in Primary Care January 2008*, unless there is a clear indication not to.

The Select Advisory Committee on Antibacterial Resistance (SACAR) and previously the Standing Medical Advisory Committee (SMAC) provide the following advice on antibacterial prescribing[1]:
No prescribing of antibiotics for simple coughs and colds
No prescribing of antibiotics for viral sore throats
Limit prescribing for uncomplicated cystitis to three days in otherwise fit women
Limit prescribing of antibiotics over the telephone to exceptional cases.

Consider alternative strategies to prescribing antibiotics:
> *Deferred prescriptions* are now increasingly seen as a legitimate method of reducing antibiotic usage (BMJ 2003; 327:1361-2). A systematic review (Br J Gen Prac 2003; 53:871-877) found a *consistent reduction in antibiotic usage when deferred prescriptions were issued*
> Those *patients given antibiotics are more likely to re-consult.*
> Studies have shown that it is possible *to avoid one repeat attendance for every nine patients not given an antibiotic.*
> Consider and suggest *routine analgesia to manage symptoms*

APPENDIX 9

Organising and Running a Journal Club for Non-Medical Prescribers

In this appendix, which refers to Chapter 9, an example is offered as to how to use a framework to build a search strategy to guide evidence based practice in relation to a clinical question.

9:1 Example of how to use PICO to build a search strategy

Example of how to use PICO to build a search strategy (reproduced with permission from Julia Hayes, Oxford Brookes University Library Services):

Patient scenario

Alice is a 70-year-old patient who was referred to the memory clinic 2 months ago by her GP with ongoing memory problems. Her GP assessed her mini-mental state as 19/30 and your previous assessment confirmed this. She has had a CT scan since your last assessment, which was consistent with a diagnosis of Alzheimer's disease.

At the last appointment you had raised the possibility of this diagnosis and some of the treatment options available. Following that appointment you wanted to undertake a search to find out how effective drug therapy is in the management of Alzheimer's disease.

How would you **PICO** this?

P- Patients with Alzheimer's disease
I- Drug therapy
C- Placebo
O- Improved or maintained cognitive function.

How could you formulate this into an answerable question in order to build a search strategy?

In patients with Alzheimer's disease does drug therapy compared with placebo improve or maintain cognitive function?
Which are the key words from the question?
Alzheimer's disease, drug therapy, placebo, cognitive function

Alzheimer* disease	Drug Therap*	Manag*
Neurological Disorder*	Drug*	Treat*
Dementia	Medicat*	
Elderly Mental Health	Psychiatric Disorders – Drug Therap*	

Think about the Boolean operators and symbols you are going to use (AND, OR, *?).
Alzheimer* Disease OR Neurological Disorder* OR Dementia OR Elderly Mental Health AND Drug Therap* AND improve* OR maintan* mental health

PubMed (MEDLINE)

To search PubMed

PubMed has extensive guidelines on how to effectively search the database available on its site, which are accessible from this link: This includes clinical queries, which will search for specific therapies.
http://www.nlm.nih.gov/bsd/disted/pubmed.html

BNI:

In the default search box (Advanced Ovid Search) do 3 separate searches and then connect them using Search History.

Do one search for:

Alzheimer* Disease OR Neurological Disorder* OR Dementia OR Elderly Mental Health

Do a second search for:

Drug therap* OR Drug* OR Medicat* OR Psychiatric Disorders Drug Therap*

Do a third search for:

Manag* OR Treat*

Click on the Search History link (the link is in the blue box above the search box).

This should show you the three searches that you have just run and will show you how many results you got for each of those searches.

To combine the 3 searches together using the AND operator:

- Tick the boxes next to each of the 3 searches
- Click on the AND button.

This will combine your 3 searches together.

You could apply a limit to your search to narrow it down further. (Limit options (such as limiting by publication year) are available underneath the search box).

You may also find that by looking through this initial set of results that there is a particular drug, or a particular aspect of drug therapy that you would like to focus your search on. You could then revise your search strategy to narrow your search down further.

Click on display to look at your results.

CINAHL

Enter your first search string in the first search box (Alzheimer* Disease OR Neurological Disorder* OR Dementia OR Elderly Mental Health).

The next string is automatically connected by the AND operator.

In the second box enter your second search string (Drug therap* OR Drug* OR Medicat* OR Psychiatric Disorders Drug Therap*).

The next string is automatically connected by the AND operator.

In the third search box enter your third search string (Manag* OR Treat*).

Click on search.

This brings up quite a lot of results – so you could apply a limit (e.g. by publication type or publication year. Limit options are displayed under the search box). You may also find that by looking through this initial set of results that there is a particular drug, or a particular aspect of drug therapy that you would like to focus your search on. You could then revise your search strategy to narrow your search down further.

COCHRANE

In the default search box

Do one search for:

Alzheimer* Disease OR Neurological Disorder* OR Dementia OR Elderly Mental Health

Do a second search for:

Drug therap* OR Drug* OR Medicat* OR Psychiatric Disorders Drug Therap*

Do a third search for:

Manag* OR Treat*

Click on the search history link underneath the default search box.

You will notice that your three searches have been given numbers (#1, #2, #3).

In the Search box enter #1 and #2 and #3.

This will combine the 3 searches together with the AND operator.

Again, you may need to apply a limit to your search to narrow down the results further.

Cochrane displays your results by publication type – e.g. systematic reviews, clinical trials. Systematic reviews are all full text on Cochrane.

9:2   Acknowledgements

We are indebted to Oxford Brookes University Library Services for their support in developing this example.

Index

absorption of medicines, 98
accountability
    and non-medical prescribing, 7, 21
    to employers, 12–13
    see also clinical governance
action learning and reflection, 83–93
    benefits, 84–6, 91
    facilitation, 87–8
    organisational requirements, 86
    practical experiences, 88–90
    putting into practice, 87–91
administration of medicines
    against prescriptions, 40, 180
    guidelines, 10
    loading doses, 101
    and therapeutic monitoring, 101
adverse drug reactions, 41, 103–4, 181–2
    see also errors and incidents
agonists, 102
Allied Health Professionals, 6–7, 50, 175
annual reviews, 41, 182
antagonists, 102
appraisal
    and CPD monitoring, 24–7
    tools, 24–6
appraisal of research *see* research reviews
Association of British Pharmaceutical
    Industry (ABPI), 23
audit
    and action learning, 91, 92
    and identification of learning needs, 24

bias, 135–6
bile, 100
blended learning
    background and policy contexts,
        67–9
    defined, 65
    planning activities, 71–4
    problems and solutions, 74–5
    resources and tools, 75–9
blogs, 65, 75–6
BMJ Learning, 78
British National Formulary (BNF), 4
building community, 118–20

care plans *see* clinical management plans
categorisation of drugs, 4
cellular transport, 102
chiropodists
    numbers, 50
    and supplementary prescribing, 6–7
clinical governance, 33–4, 42, 44
    tools to support CPD, 153–61
    see also accountability
clinical management plans (CMPs),
    6, 35, 163
    contents, 37–8
    policy frameworks, 172–3
clinical trials, appraisal studies, 129–37
Code of Conduct, 21
commissioning arrangements, 53, 59–60
'Community Practitioner Formulary Nurse
    Prescribers', 4–5
    numbers, 50
'community practitioner nurse prescribing',
    4–5
    see also nurse prescribing
competency frameworks, 10, 11, 69–70
conferences and study days, 23, 54
confidence issues, 19–20
Connecting for Health, 69, 70
Consultation MLX-3338, 6
continuing education, 182–4
    cf. CPD, 18
Core Learning Unit Programmes, 68
CPD (continuing professional
    development), 41
    background and organisational
        importance, 17–18
    employer responsibilities, 11–12, 18–19,
        21–2, 192–4
    in general practice, 215–30
    identifying opportunities, 23–4
    implementation difficulties, 22–3
    monitoring and appraisal, 24–7
    prescribing knowledge sources, 54
    resources and funding, 27–8, 57–9
    role of appraisal, 24
    role of commissioning, 59–60
    role of professional accountability, 12–13

235